Hand To Hand Basal Implantology

OrangeBooks Publication

1st Floor, Rajhans Arcade, Mall Road, Kohka, Bhilai, Chhattisgarh - 490020

Website: **www.orangebooks.in**

© Copyright, 2024, Author

All rights reserved. No part of this book may be reproduced, stored in a retrieval system, or transmitted, in any form by any means, electronic, mechanical, magnetic, optical, chemical, manual, photocopying, recording or otherwise, without the prior written consent of its writer.

First Edition, 2024

ISBN: 978-93-6554-030-7

HAND TO HAND BASAL IMPLANTOLOGY

DR. ARPIT OZA
DR. HETVI TANNA

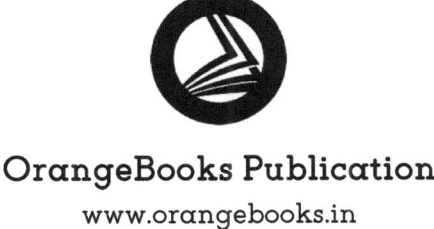

OrangeBooks Publication
www.orangebooks.in

Preface

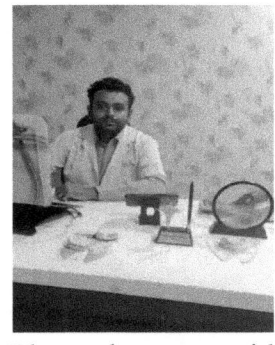

Dr. Arpit Oza

MDS (Periodontist & Oral Implantologist)

There is no doubt for dentists to evolve themselves. So, I compile each chapter in context to believe in fundaments of hierarchy of basal implantology. It is easy to read and approach. The dynasty is a proportion in practice. This book is helpful to build strategy to learn basal implantology.

Please do concern ideas, suggestions, and motivation at appes2222007@gmail.com

Acknowledgment

First of all I am thankful to almighty God for being kind in every moment of my life.as we age we learn to appreciate ourselves for our kind. So, I am very grateful to almighty for Salvation and motivation in my life.

I would like to thank my parents for their constant support in my education and my creativity. They blessed me through their internal vision. I am grateful to have such parents who showered me with their possibilities.

I would like to thank my elder brother for giving the best advice, which has made my life more fruitful. Preaching is considered by God, but for that, we must have patience.

I would like to thank my beloved wife for revealing my potential and possibilities through her insights into my work. She is truly generous, through n through with her kindness.

I would like to thank Dr.Hetvi Tanna for elevating my vision to the new level with her ideas and possibilities . The facts remain but ideologies evolve .

Content

1. Introduction 1
2. Review of Literature 5
3. Rationale & Classification Basal Implant 11
4. Comparison OF Crestal With Basal Dental Implants 21
5. Indications & Contarindications of Basal Implant 23
6. Advantages & Disadvantages of Basal Implant 24
7. Case Report 25
8. Discussion 39
9. Summary And Conclusion 48
10. Bibliography 49

Introduction

In recent years, patient demands for immediate restoration and desires to eliminate the compromised esthetics, function, discomfort and inconvenience associated with traditional two stage implant procedures have fostered interests in early and immediate loading. Literature on immediate loading of a single tooth restoration tends to be short term with occlusal contact, that ranges from unspecified, or non-occluding to lightly or fully occluding. [1,2]

Treatment plans which include several steps of surgery are less attractive or simply rejected because the costs of lost work-time and travelling adds up to the total costs of treatment. In addition, the willingness to wait for the healing of the bone and to suffer a multi-step treatment plan and especially to accept collateral damages in bone donor regions is rapidly vanishing. This all advocates for the use of basal implants as one of the options to avoid augmentations, bone transplants, distractions and similar additional operations. [3,4]

Placement of root form implants in the atrophic regions of the jaw especially in posterior mandible and below the maxillary sinus can be difficult and often impossible. Adjunctive procedures for enlarging the bone volume increase the risks of overall treatment and they reduce thereby the predictability. [5,6,7]

Patient who typically may be turned down due to smoking or periodontal involvement are good candidates for basal implants[1,8].

Basal implants provide transmission of masticatory forces not to the cancellous bone as conventional cylindrical or screw form implants, but to the stable cortical bone[9]. These implants are placed bicortically and transosseously and at least one base plate is anchored in the basal cortical bone. The primary amount of crestal and spongeous bone is unimportant for this implant pattern to become fixed[10,11]. They utilize basal bone areas free of infection and resorption, which are not necessarily located near the masticatory surfaces, therefore, are also well suited for placement immediately after extractions [12,13]. This rationale stems from orthopaedic surgery and from experience that cortical areas are needed in the structure, therefore are resistant against resorption and reconstitute itself easily[14,15]. At the same time load bearing capacities of cortical bone are many times higher than those of spongious bone[16,17]. They have a functional applicability in bone tissue with a low quality, where other type of implants fail [11].

It is understood today, that basal implants undergo a dual mechanism of integration: ring areas in direct contact with the native bone show primary integration, though osteonal remodeling also occurs. Empty slot areas (the void space left after osteotomy and insertion) fills with woven bone first and undergoes a remodeling later on[18,19]. This dual integration also allows placement of basal implants right into extraction sockets of teeth, cavities and empty spaces left after cystectomies or granulation tissue removals, or even be applicated trans-sinusally[20]. Basal implants have long being used in ridges with quantitative and/or qualitative poor bone and avoid augmentations and reopening with immediate function.[21]

In crestal implantology, sterile insertion is a major requirement, since no gap is left for suppuration. Pre-existing residual osteitis within the bone or micro-organisms introduced during the insertion, can bring treatment with crestal implants to an end very quickly. BOI implants by contrast are highly resistant to infection[22,23].

The BOI's procedure is not only the fastest and safest treatment procedure today in dental implantology, it is also the cheapest.

There is a long tradition of combining basal implants with the same or other implant systems or with stable teeth. Available data on use of these implants for single tooth replacement is minimal. Professionals who use basal implants continue to discuss whether to do so or not, which should be validated with such data analysis as reported in this study.[24]

Basal implants are endosseous aids to create osseointegrated points of retention for fixed or removable dentures. These types of implants are not only differentiated by the way they are inserted and even the way forces are transmitted. Rather, the more substantial differences lie in the planning and execution of periodontal &prosthodontic care in the post-insertion treatment regime. For this reason, the literature on basal implants has introduced the terms "Orthopaedic Technique" and "Orthopaedic Implant"[1] to mark a clear distinction between them and the well-known term "Dental Implant".[10]

Basal implants employ the basal cortical portion of the jaws for implant retention.[13] These implants are uniquely and specifically designed for the sole purpose of gaining anchorage from the basal cortical bone and have gone through several changes and modifications in the past several decades. The modern basal implant has a sophisticated yet simple design, surgical protocol and is a prosthetic friendly system. These properties have led several practitioners around the globe to include basal implantology in their practices and so far, this system has delivered fairly successful results.[12,14]

Basal implants were developed primarily for immediate use as well as for use in the atrophied jawbone. They can also be applied where very little vertical bone is present, while the supply of horizontal bone is still sufficient, even if these quantities are not contiguous such as in the sinus region.[15]

There are no difficult or impossible cases for implantologists familiar with basal implants, and their use leads in all cases straight forward to the desired treatment result. With basal implants, the regions of load transmission and the place of bacterial attack do not coincide; no masticatory forces need to be transmitted to the bone via vertical aspects of the implant; the positive retention in the bone is created in the cortical bone region. The typical objective of treatments including basal implants is a fixed restoration with multiple teeth per jaw. Optionally, removable dentures may be inserted as well, as long as enough basal implants are splinted by rigid connectors (i.e., bars).[6] Single crowns are primarily realized on internal or single-unit BOI implants. They may be loaded immediately only in favorable situations. As the use of BOI implants can help avoid risky and expensive bone augmentation procedures, these implants are the therapy of first choice in moderately or severely atrophied jaws as well as in those cases, where immediate loading or cheaper treatments are desired by the patients.[1,6]

With basal implants, load transmission is supposed to occur primarily, and initially exclusively, within the basal aspect of the implant, far away from the site of bacterial infection from the oral cavity. All aspects of the implant are smoothly polished.

Several basal implant systems with different platforms are available today; internal systems that can be secured against rotation and that have an internal screw connection and external systems that do not have a rotation-protected external thread. With basal implants, the terms internal and external thus refers to the thread and not as with crestal implants to the type and position of the surfaces that protect against rotation. By design, the mucosal penetration areas are considerably smaller with external systems than with internal systems. Whether or not this results in different degrees of resistance to infection (countable as losses / time unit) has not been examined.

Examining the status of the peri-implant bone with a probe is considered malpractice with basal implants, as no osseointegration is required on the vertical aspect of the implant anyway for permanent function of the implant. The path of insertion of the vertical aspect of the implants can no longer be determined postoperatively, and the positions of the horizontal disk suspensions are unknown. For those two reasons probing may yield false results. On the other hand, probing may carry pathogens into the depth of the interfacial region that is filled with non-irritant connective tissue at a time, when there is little chance of suppuration left. Callus formation and the maturation of the callus in the slot areas are endangered through probing. Facultative pathogens can be transported to an environment that is normally inaccessible to them and cause great damage. In particular, the maxillary sinus area may be contaminated by germs of oral origin by simple probing, if bone height is reduced or if a trans-sinus implant insertion was performed.

Probing around basal implants is therefore contraindicated and potentially dangerous. The same considerations show that rinses and any medication down along the threaded pins and under pressure are contraindicated. This is because ahead of the medication, liquid contaminated with pathogens is pressed into the deep without any control. The direction of flow is deleteriously inverted, resulting in infectious osteolysis which is otherwise a rare occurrence.[16]

The pressure of forced medication down along the threaded pins applied by the treatment provider and his syringe is greater by a factor than the internal pressure of the bone or soft tissues, so that this procedure will almost invariably result in massive introduction of germs and the spread of infection, which may become chronic. A similar effect is observed if dental restorations are seated loosely on individual implants for a prolonged time period (months or years) and the continuous relative movement of the abutment and crown creates a chronic submucosal inoculation with debris and pathogens. Here too, inoculation pressure is higher than internal tissue pressure, resulting in repeated inversion of the direction of flow and increasing osteolysis due to the measures taken by the body to fight infections. With basal implants, there are normally no funnel or cratershaped areas of bone collapse anyway, as the cortical bone closes as part of the healing process and no infection can be transported into the depth of the bone along the smooth threaded pins. Exceptions may occur if there is functionally related massive vertical bone growth along the threaded pin.[17]

Surprisingly, bone growth is in some cases unfavorable, but this is explained by the fact that bone growth will cause colonized intraoral areas of the implant to be relocated to submucosal or enossal regions. The proper therapy in these cases consist invariably in creating local drainage around the vertical implant part. With integrated basal implants, infection originating in the oral cavity would not normally be expected to spread enossally, for as long as the implants are not mobile to the extent that they can be intruded. Infections can be caused by food retention or impaction or as a consequence of vertical bone growth. However, unlike with crestal implants, they do not spread intraosseously but submucosally. The latter may result in infected vertical parts if the implants are submerged below the mucosal level over time, eliminating the necessary gateway for suppuration as the area of penetration is closed with scar tissue. Any inflammation of this type will spread just like a submucosal abscess and is treated in the same way. It is recommended to make generous incisions to open the abscess. The mucosal area immediately adjacent to the threaded pin can be excised by electrosurgery. In rare cases, reduction osteotomies or the replacement of implants will be required if vertical bone growth becomes excessive.[17,18]

Bicortical screws (BCS) are also considered basal implants, because they transmit masticatory loads deep into the bone, usually into the opposite cortical bone, while full osseointegration along the axis of the implant is not a prerequisite. BCS provide at least initially some elasticity and they are not prone to peri-implantitis due to their polished surface and thin mucosal penetration diameter.

Review of Literature

The first enossal implant design that relied on a lateral insertion path and capitalized on the stability of both the inner and outer cortical bone was devised in Italy (FP Spahn, Personal Communication)[20]. The disk and vertical threaded pin were inserted separately in this design, the latter through an additional vertical drill hole. Finally both components were connected with a screw. The technological means of single unit titanium implants of adequate size were not available at that time.

The first single unit implant was developed and used by Jean-Marc Julliet (1972)[14]. This design was available in one size and offered no basal plate resilience. The scope of indications for this design was limited to the areas where the basal plate reached both cortical structures, so that its use was essentially confined to the anterior segments of either jaw.

The original implant design by Lobello was based on inserting two separate components, whereas the design by Julliet featured a welded joint between the threaded pin and basal plate[21].

In 1991, Scortecci et al. published a retrospective study on the clinical outcomes of his Diskimplant system. In the years 1979-1989, a total of 5,848 implants had been inserted, 590 of which had to be removed because the disc diameters were too small or the threaded pins were too short. Also another factor was that the original discs were not perforated at all[1,2].

With Scortecci's development of standardized cutters for implant beds, lateral implantology ultimately became an option even in the hands of less skillful surgeons. Therefore Scortecci is rightly regarded as one of the ***"Founding Father's of Lateral implantology"*** [2,3].

Ihde and Spahn laid the foundation for basal osseointegration, by applying for a patent on the first elastic implant design, thus turning away in theory and practice from the rather mechanistic theory of crestal implants and rigid bone-implant prosthetic systems[3,4].

The basal implants were configured to match the anatomical shape of the jawbone and the crestal plate was positioned in a more resilient position than the basal plate. By virtually eliminating the risk of crestal osteolysis in the maxilla, this development can be regarded as a milestone in the history of BOI27. At the same time, load transmission in the area of the crestal plate was confined to the palatal bone, which appeared to be much better suited for this task in terms of structure, resorption tendency and blood supply compared to the vestibular bone. Ihde and Spahn in a collaborative effort developed implants that behaved elastically within the bone, allowing resilience of the threaded pin5,7. This enabled the transmission of unequal loads on the base plate. The base plate was designed to be more rigid than the crestal plate. Hence, the larger portion of chewing forces was transmitted to the lower plate while the crestal plate provided stabilization.

Asymmetrical BOI implant design, first described in 2000, was capable of compensating for the centrifugal resorption of the mandible, while the bone cavities for insertion could still be prepared with rotationally symmetrical instruments25. This design allows managing both the centripetal resorption of the upper jaw and as well as with centrifugal resorption of the lower jaw. The idea of basal, wide-area support for implants was taken up by many developers around the same point. The resolution of situations in which insufficient bone volume was available was what gave rise to various ideas. Only Julliet (1972), Scortecci (1985) and Ihde (from 1998) ever turned their ideas into successfully marketable and clinically practical products[17].

Ihde and Mutter performed a retrospective case series of 275 BOI implants in 228 patients over a period of five years. Molars were replaced with BOI implants in combination with natural abutments. Osseointegration was achieved in 254 implants at follow-up. Fifteen implants were lost. This study demonstrates that basal implants work well in combination with natural abutments.

Donsimoni et al performed a retrospective case series evaluating 1352 consequitive basalimplants placed over a 10 year period in 234 circular bridges. Osseointegration was achieved in97% of cases.

Gerard Scortecci (1999)[16], conducted a clinical trial over a 41 month period where 783 titanium implants (627 laterally inserted disk implants, with or without 156 axially inserted implants) were placed in 72 consecutive patients with completely edentulous maxillae using an immediate loading protocol. He concluded that immediate loading of laterally inserted disk-design implants with a fixed, functional prosthesis is a safe and reliable method for management of completely edentulous maxillae. The initial bucco-palatal cortical anchorage achieved with these implants ensures sufficient stability for osseointegration, and lateral insertion technique makes them suitable for seating in atrophic maxillae.

Sigmar Kopp (2007)[16], presented a report on the outcomes of using a basal implant design for treating patients especially with poor quality and quantity of bone under immediate load conditions. Out of the 302 implants placed in 88 patients, 13 implants failed during follow-up period giving an overall survival rate of nearly 96%. Basal implants used for single tooth replacement showed the lowest survival rate (90.9%), but this was the result of specific overload. The highest loss rate was found in the first days and the survival rate was found to increase by time in situ to 100% for 3 years and more.

Sigmar Kopp (2007)[17], showed an example of a patient with congenital hypodontia, who had thin bone ridges due to the absence of adequate growth stimuli. The transosseous installation of basal implants and their cortical anchorage leads to fast rehabilitation and high aesthetic results.

Henri Diederich (2007)[6], adopted a two-stage prosthetic protocol to be appropriate if teeth are extracted in anterior maxilla. Due to prior extraction of several residual teeth, pronounced bone remodeling and soft tissue recontouring is expected. This necessitates readaptation of the tissue side of the bridge after 4 months.

Sigmar Kopp (2007)[18], found that basal implants can be used immediately after extraction, even in massive periodontal involved cases. By use of BOI, just one session is needed for teeth extraction, implant placement, and immediate loadable bridge insertion. A functionally balanced occlusion can be achieved on by installation of circular bridges on 4 implants. The thin vertical shaft is smooth and has no direct load transmitting function to the bone, giving no retention to plaque or calculus. So BOI is periodontal preventive designed and practically proved.

Sigmar Kopp (2007)[23], showed by his study that, basal implants themselves are safe and effective when used without combination with crestal implants.

Henri Diederich (2008)[5], discussed an approach of implant treatment in a patient with pronounced atrophy and concluded that immediate loading with a fixed restoration could be offered and successfully implemented with the help of BOI implants and tuberopterygoid screws despite an inadequate bone volume in the vertical and horizontal planes.

Ihde et al. (2008)[13], developed a model that accurately represented the interface between bone and basal implants throughout the healing process and applied it to the biological scenario of changing load distribution in a basal implant system over time through finite element analysis, using multiple models with changing bone-implant contact definitions. They showed that, in upgraded models which more closely approximate the biological scenario with basal dental implant, peak von Mises stresses decreased at the implant interface; however they increased at the bone interface as a harder contact definition was modeled. Further, a shift in peak stress location was found within the implants during different contact definitions (i.e., different stagesof bone healing). In case of hard contact, the peak stress occurs above the contact surface, whereas in soft contact, the stress peak occurs in the upper part of the contact area between the bone and the vertical shaft of the implant. Only in extreme soft contact definitions, were the peak stresses found to be near the base of the implant.

Stefan Ihde (2008)[22], in his case report showed that basal implants are an excellent alternative in patients with implant failures, to provide a new implant(s), in lieu of prosthesis and allow the patient to return to normal masticatory function with little or no delay.

Sigmar Kopp and Wilfried Kopp (2008)[22,25], described the immediate placement of basal implants even in the infected extraction sockets under real immediate prosthetic loading conditions as a safe and effective way of treatment. He concluded that waiting for healing of the sockets after extractions does not improve the general success rate of BOI and BCS (basal compressionscrew) implants and may be generally avoided.

Stefan Ihde (2009)[19,] discussed the value of using basal implants and the differences that exist between basal implants and crestal implants in peri-operative status, infection around integrated implants, load transmission and replacement of failing implants. He concluded that, the technique of basal implantology solves all the problems connected with conventional (crestal) implantology.

Konstantinovic et al. (2010)[28], reported a case of a patient who underwent facial reconstruction with nasal epithesis anchored on basal (disk) implants after ablation of midface squamous cell carcinoma. After an unloaded osseointegration phase of three months, all implants appeared well integrated according to radiological criteria and clinical stability. The case was followed up for 18 months and there were no signs of recurrence of the tumor, nor any complications related to the implants. The authors concluded that disk implants that were applied in this case present an excellent alternative, particularly in cases with minimal available bone, resulting in reduced complications in elderly oncological patients.

Borak L et al.(2010)[10], in the first of their biomechanical study of single and double disk implants, described the mechanical interaction between the implant and the bone tissue in terms of the quality of bone tissue, the osseointegration level, and the character of the implant anchorage. They analyzed the cranioapical displacement of the implant and the strain intensity in cancellous bone. They described three variants of anchorage within the bone :

Variant A - mechanical interaction between implant disk, inner and outer cortical bone.

Variant B - interaction with outer cortical bone only.

Variant C - implant disk is smaller than space between outer and inner cortical bone wheretherein is interaction with cancellous bone only.

They concluded that only Variant A and the double disk implant guarantees the possibility of immediate loading of the implant after the application regardless of the quality of bone tissue. Also despite a negligible difference in displacements in variants A and B, the difference in strain intensity is significant.

Marcian P et al. (2010)[11], in second part of the same study, focussed on the stress-strain analysis (and toleralability) of disk implants as loaded during the masticatory process.

Adel.A. Chidac (2010)[1], described the various surgical techniques to avoid a sinus lift procedure and showed that disk implants are a favourable alternative to sinus elevation and bone augmentation other than tilted implants and tuberosity implants.

Scortecci et al. (2010)[4], described a case of squamous cell carcinoma of the oral cavity managed with ablative surgery, mandibular reconstruction with a fibula free flap, and implant placement during the same session. They concluded that early functional dental rehabilitation with one step immediate loading procedure is possible provided the concepts of basal implantology are respected.

Stefan Ihde and Sigmar Kopp (2010)[20,] reviewed the available literature on basal implants and lined out a treatment concept without bone augmentation for upper jaw. They have presented simple treatment plans to avoid sinus lifts using basal implants, as almost all patients have sufficient horizontal bone naturally, even if vertical bone is missing.

Ihde et al. (2010)[21], showed that palatal and vestibular placements of basal implants may be combined to increase the primary stability of the bridge, splinting the implants under immediateload conditions.

Ihde and Konstantinovic (2011)[14], explained the four options for treating extremely atrophic posterior mandible with basal implants:

a. Infra-nerve implant placement.

b. Placement of basal implants after caudalisation of alveolar nerve and vessels.

c. Placement of basal implants in anterior part of ascending ramus of mandible.

d. Application of basal implants as sub-periosteal implant.

They concluded that these methods are a superior alternative to the traditional techniques of increasing the bone volume, such as distraction-osteogenesis and vascularized or non-vascularized bone block transplants.

Ruzov et al. (2011)[12], showed that puncturing the flaps and flipping them over the implant's head, provide the possibility for closing tightly over single-piece (lateral) basal implants. In combination with double-mattress sutures this technique allows to create a tight seal around the projection vertical part of the basal implant.

Siddharth Shah (2011)[15], showed that in severely resorbed cases of distal mandible, the implant must be placed well below the amber line (linea obliqua) for stable results. In this way the implants rest in the resorption stable bone and the success rates are high.

T. Goldman et al. (2011)[3], analysed the force transfer and stress distribution of an implant supported circular bridge with rectangular cross section bridge in the atrophied mandible and considered two different designs for the bridge in posterior mandible – a) direct straight line connection between the posterior implant in the mandible and the bridge and; b) connection between posterior implant and bridge with posterior implant designed as technical abutments. They concluded that direct straight line connection is from the biomechanic point of view, the least desirable solution for the BAST type implant, because stresses within the implant, the bridge and the bone are higher compared to prosthetic solutions where implant remains outside the lower arch.

S. Ihde et al. (2011)[7], showed the relationship between bridge core diameters, the resistance of peri-implant bone and stresses around the endosseous base plates of immediately loaded basal implants using finite element analysis and concluded that the success of a treatment with immediately loaded basal implants in strategic positioning depends strongly on the rigidity of the bridge, i.e. on the bridge-core diameter. Dimensions of 2.5x3.5 mm or more for the bridge core are required for treatment in immediate load protocols.

Rationale & Classification of Basal Implant

According to the concept of basal implantology the jaw bone comprises of two parts the tooth bearing alveolus or crestal part and the basal bone. The crestal bone is less dense in nature and is exposed to infections from tooth borne pathologies, injuries or iatrogenic factors and is therefore subject to higher rate of resorption whereas the basal bone is heavily corticated and is rarely subject to infections and resorption. It is this, i.e., the basal bone that can offer excellent support to the implants because of its densely corticated nature, at the same time the load bearing capacity of the basal bone is many times higher than that offered by the spongy crestal bone. This rationale stems from Orthopedic surgery and from the experience that cortical areas are essential, since, they are resistant to resorption, as a result basal implants are also called as Orthopaedic Implants. 27,9

Classification of Basal Implant Types Based on Morphology:
There are four basic types of basal implants available-

  I. Screw Form.
  II. Disk Form.
  III. Plate Form.
  IV. Others

Both of the types can be further categorized into-
  I. Screw Form
   a. Compression Screw Design (KOS Implant)
   b. Bi-Cortical Screw Design (BCS Implant)
   c. Compression Screw + Bi-Cortical Screw Design (KOS plus Implant)
  II. Disk Form

Basal Osseointegrated Implant (BOI) / Trans-Osseous

Implant (TOI) / Lateral Implant

1. **According to abutment connection-**
   i. Single Piece Implant.
   ii. External Threaded Connection.
   iii. Internal Threaded Connection.

    a. External Hexagon.

    b. External Octagon.

2. According to basal plate design-
    i. Basal disks with angled edges

    ii. Basal disks with flat edges also called as S-Type Implant

3. According to number of disks-
    i. Single Disk.

    ii. Double Disk.

    iii. Triple Disk.

III. Plate Form

    a. BOI-BAC Implant

    b. BOI-BAC2 Implant

IV. Other Forms

    a. TPG Implant (Tuberopterygoid).

    b. ZSI Implant (Zygoma Screw).

Morphology of basal implant:

The BOI (Basal Osseo Integrated) and BCS (Basal Cortical Screw) implant being produced today has a smooth and polished surface as it was found that polished surfaces are less prone to inflammation (mucositis, periimplantitis) than rough surfaces. The KOS and KOS Plus implants are surface treated (sand and grit blasting with subsequent acid etching), however, the implant neck is kept highly polished in KOS implant. In the KOS Plus implant, its neck and the basal cortical screw part are kept heavily polished. BOI (lateral basal implants): is inserted from the lateral aspect of the jaw bone and it requires minimum bone height of 3 mm and that means virtually every patient can be treated without bone grafting. Because bone grafting is avoided, risk groups, such as smokers and diabetics, can successfully receive these implants. Wide basal disk of the implant is stabilized into both facial as well as lingual strong cortices deep into the resorption and infection resistant zone (well deep from the crest) which guarantees safe load transmission and osseointegration. Its iso-elastic (flexible) design make it possible to connect its prosthesis to the firm and healthy natural teeth in selective cases which avoid the necessity of extraction of healthy teeth and also save the cost of the treatment. The neck of this implant can be bended to make multiple implant heads parallel for passive seating of the prosthesis and also to seat the prosthesis in the most suitable occlusion line. Masticatory load transmission is confined to the horizontal implant segments and, essentially, to the cortical bone structures.

BCS (screw basal implant): Is inserted like a conventional implant, but it transmits loads only into the opposing deep cortical bone that means virtually every patient can be treated without bone grafting. Because bone grafting is avoided, also risk groups, such as smokers and diabetics, can successfully receive these implants. Strictly cortical anchorage of the implant guarantees for safe load transmission and osseointegration. Minimal invasive implant placement (Mostly without any flap and suture) the neck of this implant also can be bended to make multiple implant heads parallel for passive seating of the prosthesis and also to seat the prosthesis in the most suitable occlusion line. These implants are also heavily polished and are flapless implants with a very small mucosal penetration diameter.

Compressive implant (KOS): Is a single-component one piece Screw type basal implants with a compression thread, it is used for multiple unit restoration with immediate loading in the upper and lower jaw, it can be used in combination with other BCS basal implants (KOS Plus Implant) and allows flap and flapless placement. The first approach relies on the compression screw principle. Screw implants of this type can result in lateral condensation of spongy bone areas. Implant stability is greatly increased by a mechanism that could be regarded as "corticalization" of the spongy bone (KOS).

Parts Of Basal Implants:

The basal implants are single piece implants in which the implant and the abutment are fused into one single piece. This minimizes the failure of implants due to interface problems, the connections which exists in conventional two and three piece implants.

Surface of the implants:

- Polished surface
- Stops bacteria and plaque from adhering to the implant neck or body.

Body of the implants:

- The thin implant body is combined with wide thread turns that enhances the vascularity around the implant and increases the bone implant contact.

Neck of the implant:

- The abutment can be bent by 15-25 degrees depending upon the length of the implant, provided the implant is placed in dense corticated bone.
- The polished surface protects the implant surface from bacterial attachment.

Location of classic and basal implants

The Classic Implants are positioned in the crestal alveolar bone , which consists of bone of less quality and it is more prone to resorption. This type of bone is lost after teeth are removed and decreases through life.

The Basal Implants are inserted into the basal bone that is less prone to bone resorption and infections. The bone is highly dense, mineralized and offers an excellent support to implants and a long lasting solution for tooth loss. The basal bone is always present throughout life.

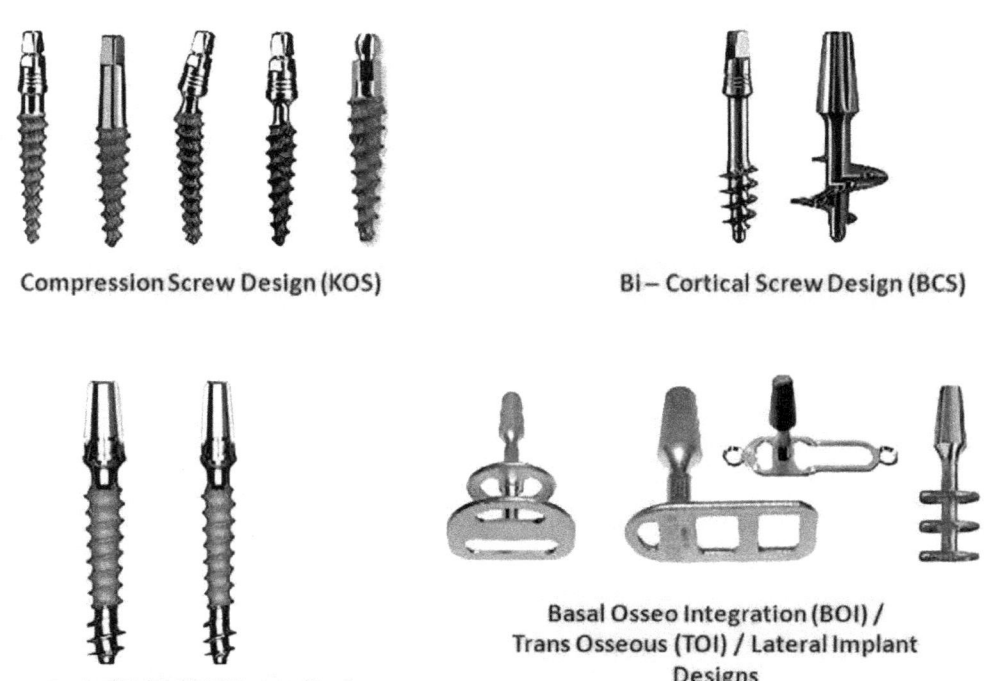

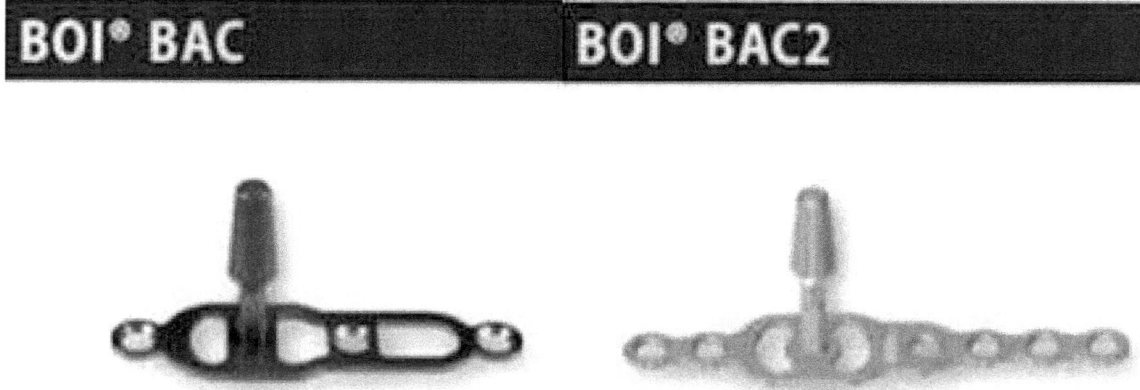

Single Piece (Monobloc) Basal Implants

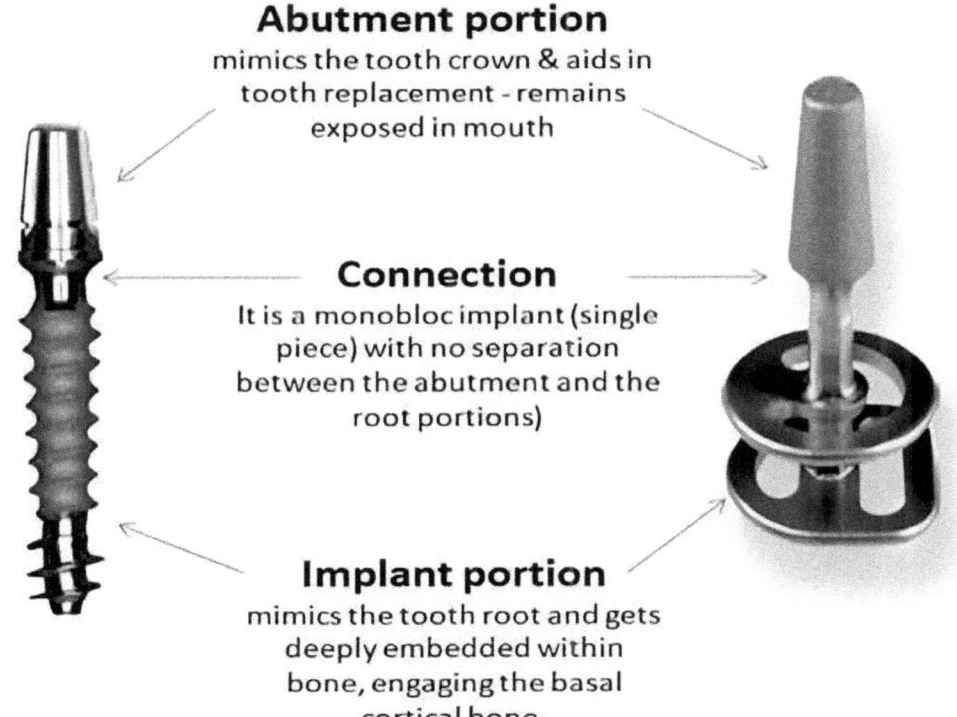

Abutment portion
mimics the tooth crown & aids in tooth replacement - remains exposed in mouth

Connection
It is a monobloc implant (single piece) with no separation between the abutment and the root portions)

Implant portion
mimics the tooth root and gets deeply embedded within bone, engaging the basal cortical bone.

Description Of Boi-Implants
Nomenclature

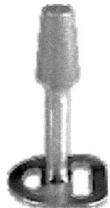

BS: Single disk BOI with antirotational cube shaped disk.

Eg: BS 7: Disk diameter 7mm

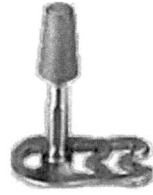

BOI – BAST

Eg: BAST 10/16: average width of 10mm and length of 16mm

Description	H	SH1	SH2	SH3	SA
BS 7	H 8	0.7-0.9			
BS 7	H 12	0.7-0.9			
BS 9	H 6	0.7-0.9			
BS 10	H 4	0.7-0.9			
BS 10	H 6	0.7-0.9			
BS 10	H 10	0.7-0.9			
BS 12	H 6	0.7-0.9			
BS 12	H 8	0.7-0.9			
BS 12	H 10	0.7-0.9			
BS 12	H 12	0.7-0.9			

DESCRIPTION	H	SH1
BAST 10/16	H 4	0.7-0.9
BAST 10/12	H 6	0.7-0.9
BAST 10/16	H 6	0.7-0.9
BAST 10/14	H 8	0.7-0.9
BAST 10/16	H 8	0.7-0.9

With cogs on flat side and may be rotated after placement.

SH2SH3SA

SH2	SH3	GD
9.5		
9.5		9.5
9.5		
9.5		

GD: maximum diameter on round side in mm

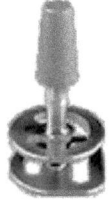

BOI – BBS

Eg: BBS 9/7: diameter of basal disk 9mm, diameter of crestal disk 7mm

DESCRIPTION	H	SH1	SH2	SH3	SA
BBS 7	H 6	0.7-0.9	0.7		3
BBS 9/7	H 6	0.7-0.9	0.7		3
BBS 9/7	H 10	0.7-0.9	0.7		3
BBS 9/7	H 8	0.7-0.9	0.7		3
BBS 10	H 4	0.7-0.9	0.7		3

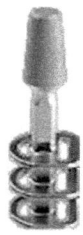

BOI – BBBS

Eg: BBBS 7: diameter of alldisks 7mm

DESCRIPTION	H	SH1	SH2	SH3	SA
BBBS 7	H 4	0.6	0.6	0.6	3
BBBS 7	H 6	0.6	0.6	0.6	3
BBBS 7	H 8	0.6	0.6	0.6	3

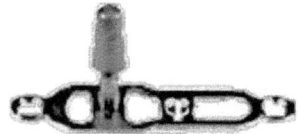

BOI - BAC

Used in severely atrophic areas, also can be used as a subperiosteal implant.

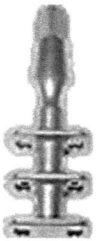

BOI - DISKOS 4T

BOI implant with asymmetric disks for use in areas with reduced mesiodistal width.

Cutters For Boi

VERTICAL CUTTER

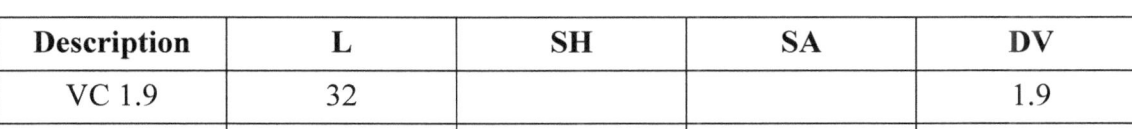

Description	L	SH	SA	DV
VC 1.9	32			1.9
VC 1.6	32			1.6

COMBINATION CUTTER

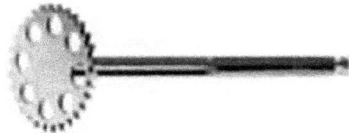

Description	L	SH	SA	DV
KC 7-4W	32	0.4		7
KC 8-4W	32	0.4		8
KCD 7-4W	32	0.4	3	7
KCXD	32	0.6	5	9

LATERAL CUTTER – Single

Description	L	SH	SA	DV
LC 7-4W	32	0.4		7
LC 7-6W	32	0.6		7
LC 7-8W	32	0.8		7
LC 8-4W	32	0.4		8
LC 9-4W	32	0.4		9
LC 9-6W	32	0.6		9
LC 9-8W	32	0.8		9
LC 9-10W	32	1.0		9

LC 10-4W	32	0.4		10
LC 10-6W	32	0.6		10
LC 10-8W	32	0.8		10
LC 12-4W	32	0.4		12
LC 12-6W	32	0.6		12

LATERAL CUTTER - Double

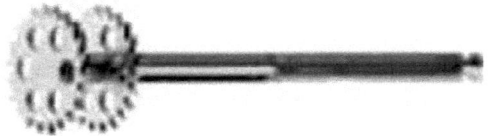

Description	L	SH	SA	DV
LCD 7-4W	32	0.4	3	7

LATERAL CUTTER - Triple

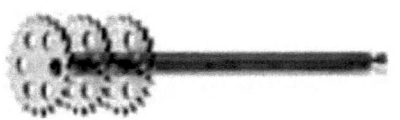

Description	L	SH	SA	DV
LCT 7-4W	32	0.4	3	7

Comparison of Crestal With Basal Dental Implants

Criteria	Crestal Implants	Basal Implants
Shape and structure	Root form – designed to imitate roots of a tooth.	The implants look like an inverted T.
Endosseous section	Screw shaped with machine / HA coated surfaces.	Flat / blade like surfaces with spaces permitting bone in growth. No one of them equipped with any kind of prepared surface for the enhancement of bone regeneration.
Technique	Insertion through crestal bone and communication with oral cavity much more than basal implants.	Insertion through lateral aspect of basal bone. Load bearing area of implant has no communication with the oral cavity.
Bone requirement	Vertical bone – both crestal and rarely a small portion of basal bone.	Basal bone is what is needed. Horizontal aspects of the bone are fully utilized along with the inner and outer cortices.
Armamentarium	A large number of Instruments are necessary for procedures.	Instrumentation relatively a lot simpler.
Bone grafting procedures	Essential in cases of deficiency in bone height. Grafting procedures give unpredictable results.	Not essential.
Bone displacement	Considerable bone substance displacement / loss occur and vary with size and length	Displace up to 60% less bone substance. Basal bone – highly

	of implant. Crestal bone is more susceptible to resorption.	resistant to resorption.
Mucosal penetration diameter	Larger. Chances of Periimplantitis, vertical bone loss, crater like bone loss and infections are relatively high.	Smaller (1.9 – 2.3 mm. only). The whole vertical implant part is polished – hence, chances of problems seen as in the case of crestal implants relatively very low.
Loading	Two piece crestal implants often require delayed loading & two surgical phases at times.	Immediate loading.
Healing	Prolonged healing time – clinically significant.	Bone healing time not clinically significant.
Masticatory forces	They act in the vertical direction along the sides of the screw structure.	Transferred to the basal plate deep into the cortical bone areas which are able to accept large loads and have great capacity for regeneration.
Applications in destructive periodontitis & after multiple extractions of teeth	Their placement in such cases is nearly impossible and success is unpredictable.	Placement of implants is very much possible and results are excellent.
Smoking patients	Failure rate is close to 100%.	Best option for smoking patients.
Controlled diabetic patients	Crestal implants have a risk of failure in cases, where there are blood sugar variations.	Blood sugar variations may not affect the survival of the implant at all.

Indications & Contarindications of Basal Implant

INDICATIONS:

1. All kinds of situations when several teeth are missing or have to be extracted.

2. When the procedure of 2-stage implant placement or bone augmentation has failed.

3. All kinds of bone atrophy i.e.,
   a. In cases of very thin ridges- i.e., deficiency of bone in buccolingual thickness.
   c. In cases of insufficient bone height.

These two situations develop due to the following reasons.
   a. Using removable dentures for so many years will resorb the bone and reduce the height available.
   b. After extraction of teeth, not replacing the teeth, living without teeth for many years will also resorb the bone.
   c. Untreated periodontal disease (especially in diabetics) will resorb the available bone.
   d. Trauma to jaw which damages not only the teeth but also the alveolar bone.

CONTRAINDICATIONS:

1. Special cases: Cases where bilateral equal mastication cannot be arranged, e.g. when chewing muscles or their innervations are partly missing (these cases may lead to problems under immediate load protocols).

2. Medical conditions: There are a number of medical conditions that preclude the placement of dental implants. Some of these conditions include: Recent myocardial infarction (heart attack) or cerebrovascular accident (stroke), Immunosuppression (a reduction in the efficacy of the immune system).

3. Medicines: A dentist will need a complete listing of all of the medicines and supplementsthat their patient takes. Drugs of concern are those utilized in the treatment of cancer, drugs that inhibit blood clotting and bisphosphonates (a class of drugs used in the treatment of osteoporosis).

Advantages & Disadvantages of Basal Implant

Advantages:

1. Safe load transmission in basal bone - Load transmission is deep in the infection free basal bone. In conventional root form implant, load transmission is near the area of bacterial attack. Cortical bone is resorption resistant due to higher mineralization.

2. Less incidence of peri-implant infections – Implant surface is polished in basal implants and also the mucosal penetration diameter is less as compared to conventional dental implants.

3. Patient's own alveolar bone is required - Basal implants require the patient's own alveolar bone and no bone augmentations are required. All patients have sufficient basal bone horizontally, even if vertically height is reduced. Also the duration of treatment is reduced as bone augmentations require certain amount of time for healing.

4. Immediate loading - Extremely good patient acceptance is obtained with basal implants as immediate loading is possible. There is no edentulous phase and immediate dentures are not required.

5. One stage procedure - Extractions and implant placement can be carried out in one appointment even if the teeth are periodontally infected.

6. Low demand for patient compliance.

Disadvantages:

1. Compromised aesthetics with single tooth replacement.

2. Skilled surgeon with sound anatomic knowledge is important to carry out successful surgery.

3. Excess sound bone reduction in cases of good bone support.

4. A phenomenon called as overload osteolysis can be seen, if load distribution is not done properly.

Case Report

Maxillary Posterior Boi Implant Placement

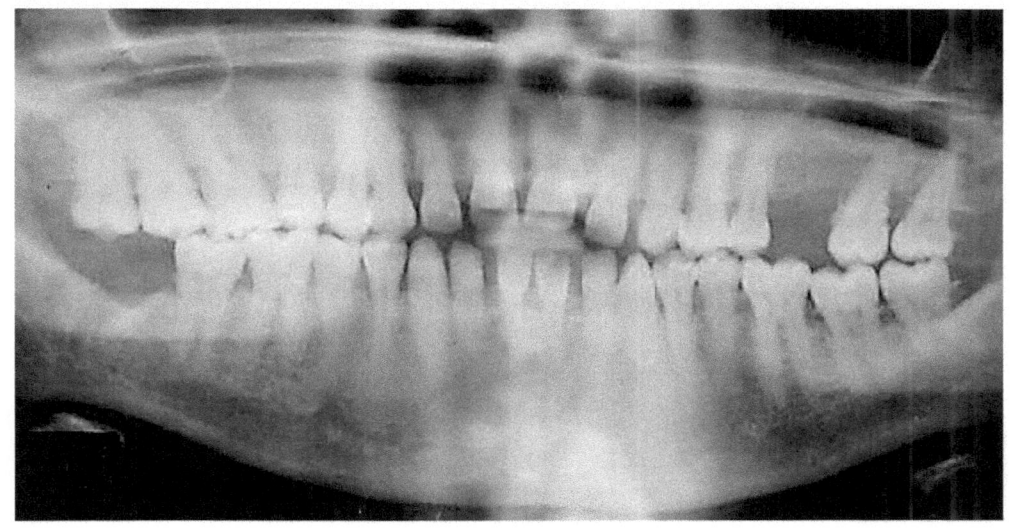

Pre-Operative Opg

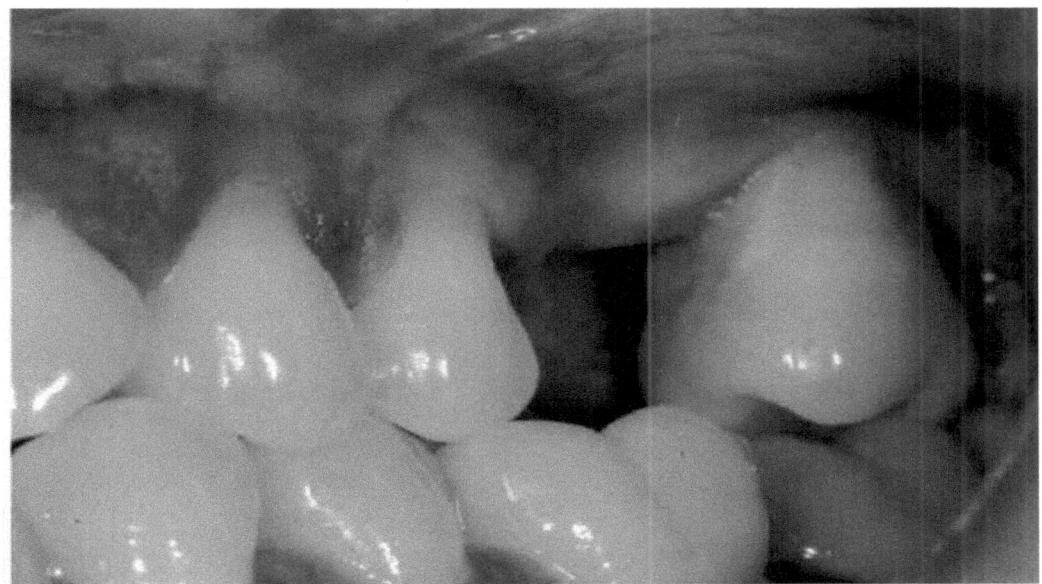

Pre-Operative Photograph

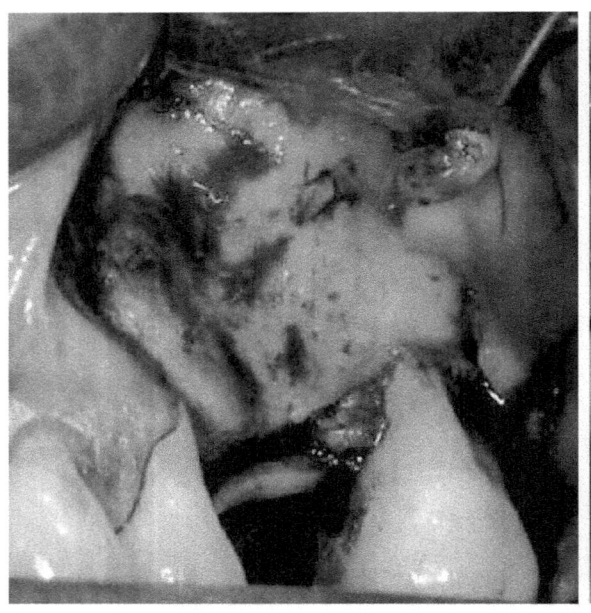
Incision And Exposure

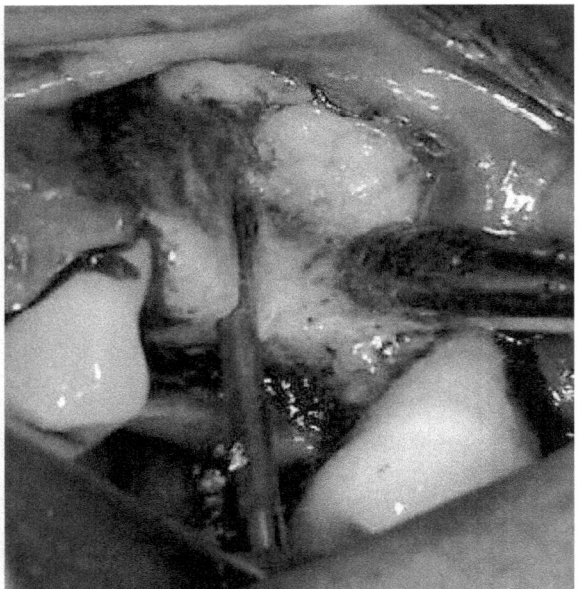
Vertical Cut Using Vc 1.6

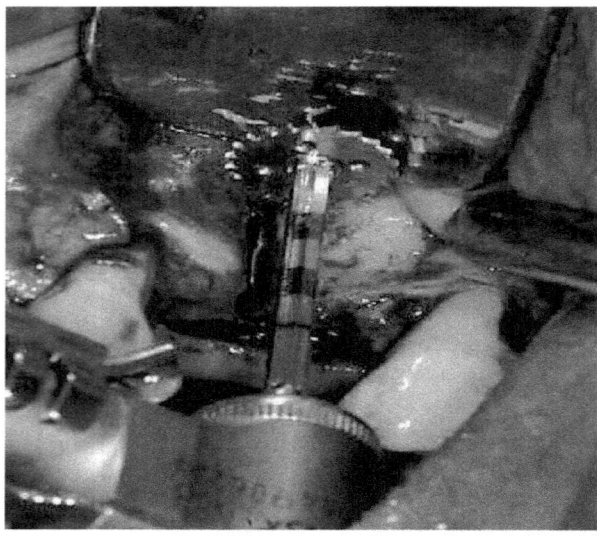
Combination Cut Using Kc 7

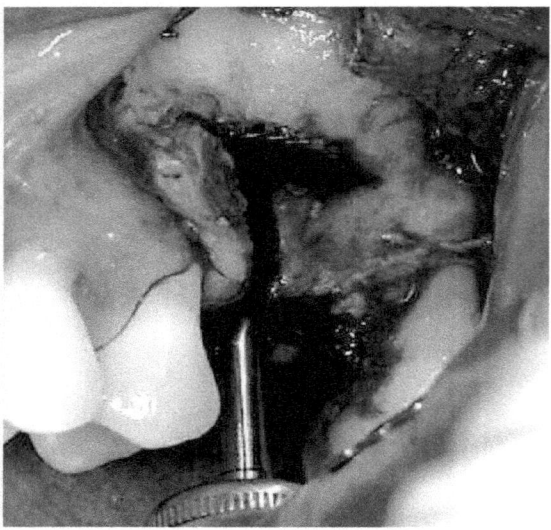
Lateral Cut Using Lc 9-6 W

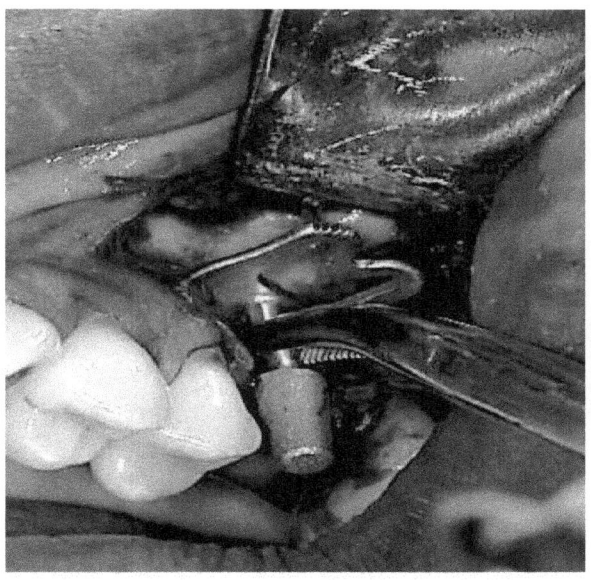

Insertion Of Boi, Bas 9/12, H6

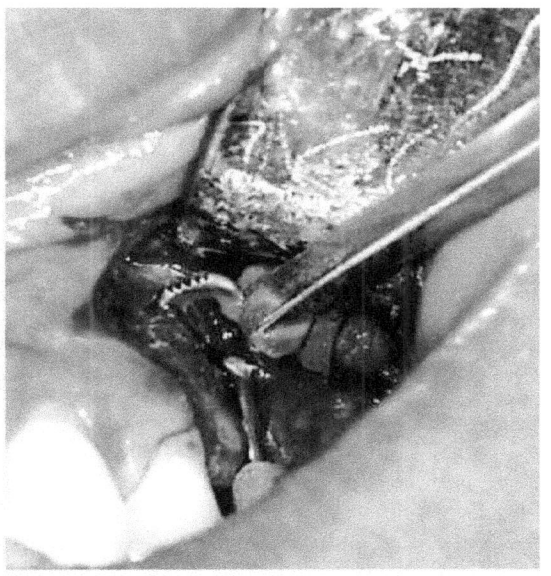

Use Of Chisel And Mallet To Tap Implant In Place

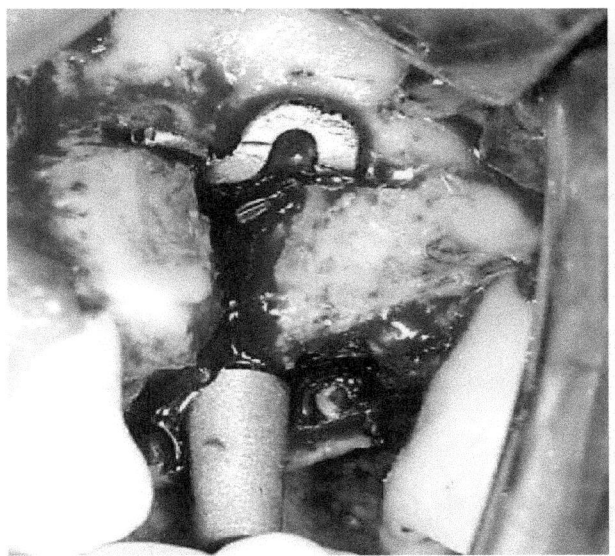

Implant Insertion Complete

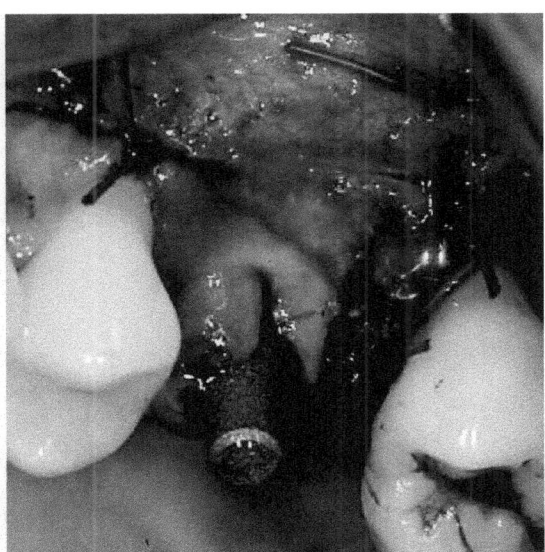

Closure

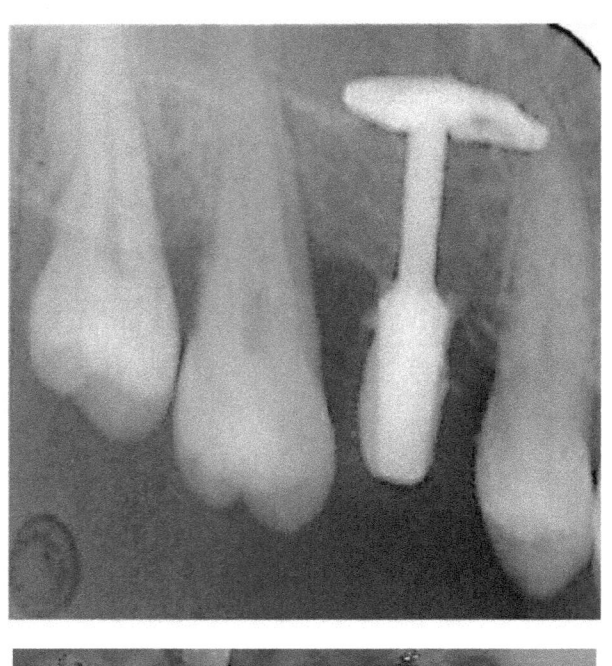

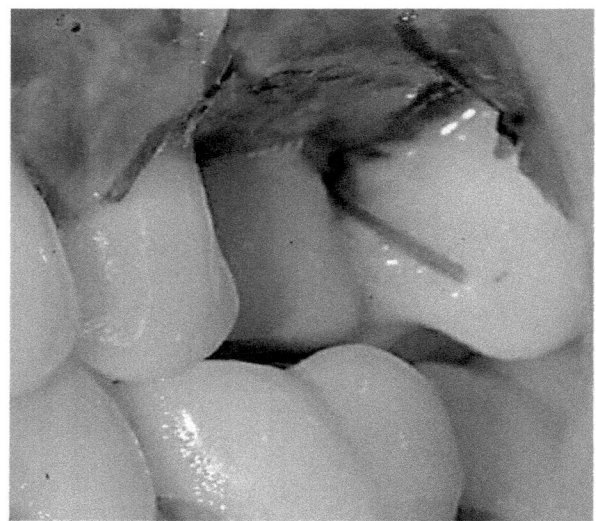

Immediate Restoration Immediate Post-Operative Iopa With Acrylic Crown

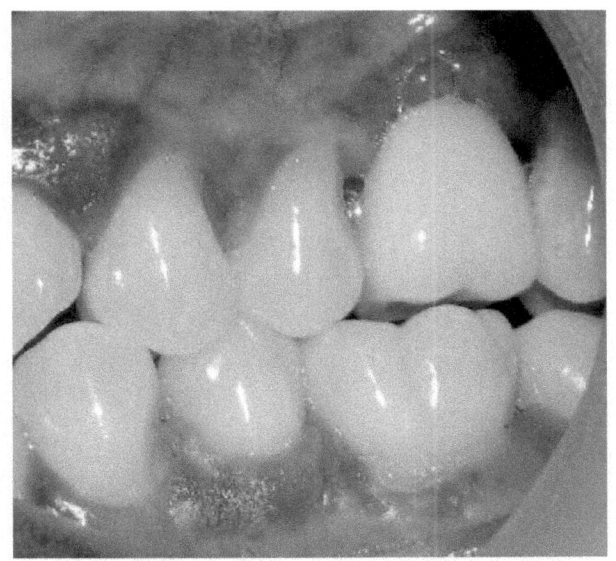
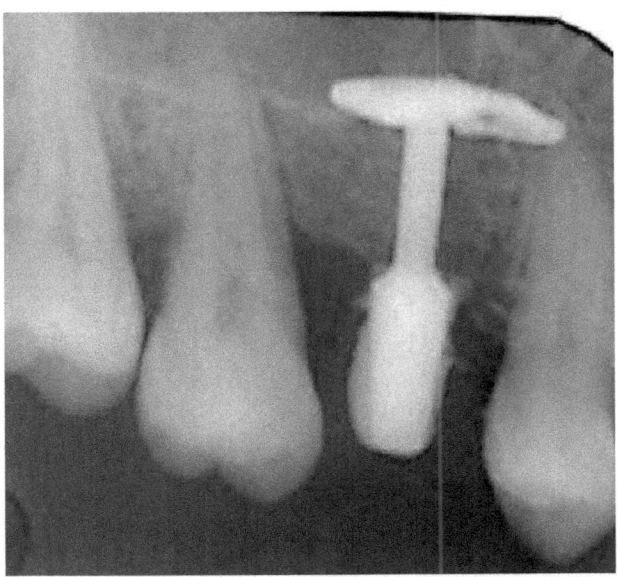

17 Months Post-Operative Iopa 17 Months Post-Operative Photograph With Ceramic Crown

Maxillary Anterior Boi Implant Placement

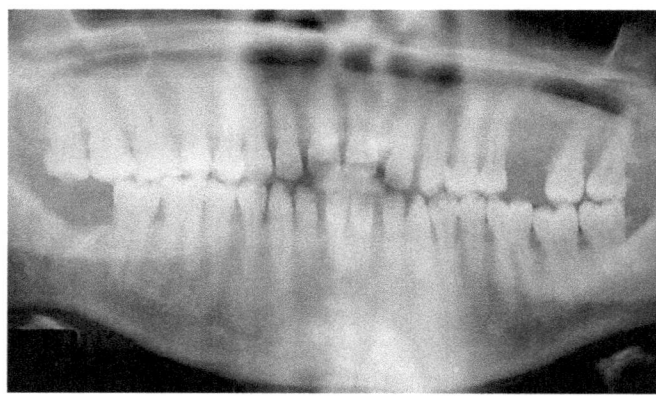

Pre-Operative Opg

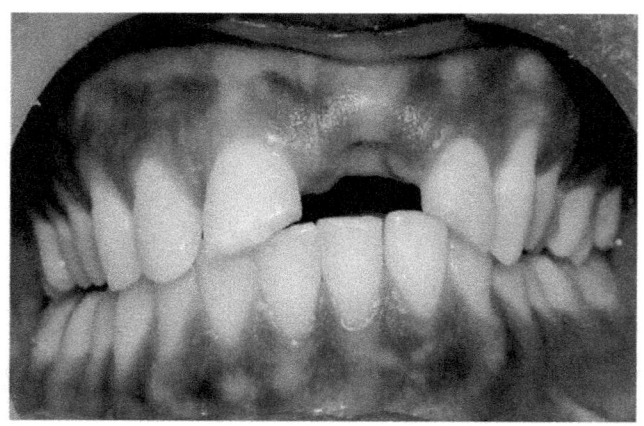

Preoperative Photograph

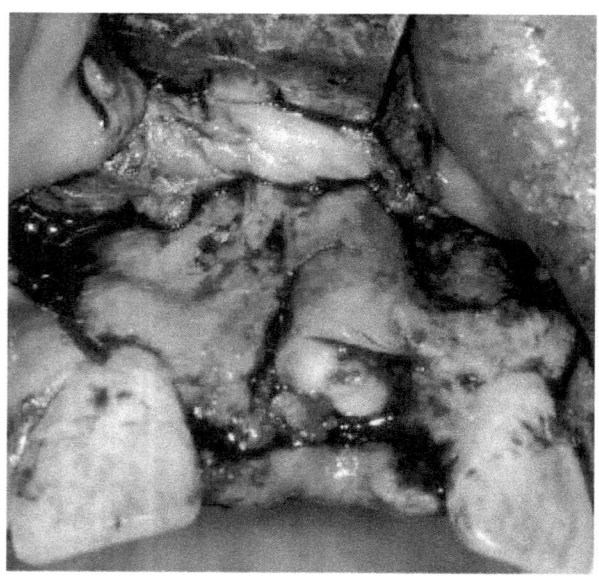
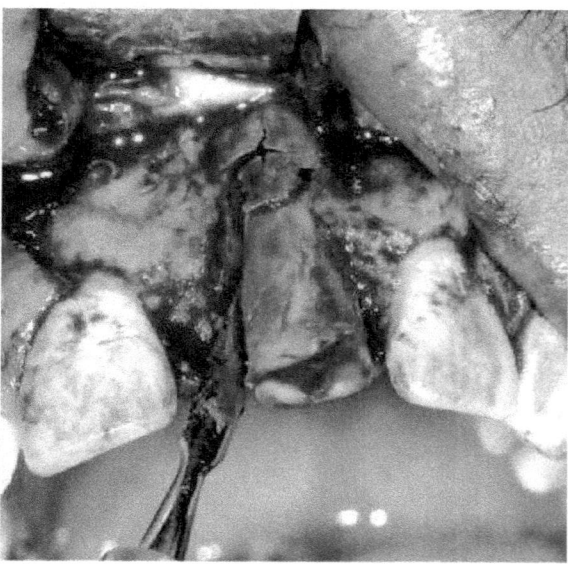

Incision And Exposure   Extraction Of Root Stump

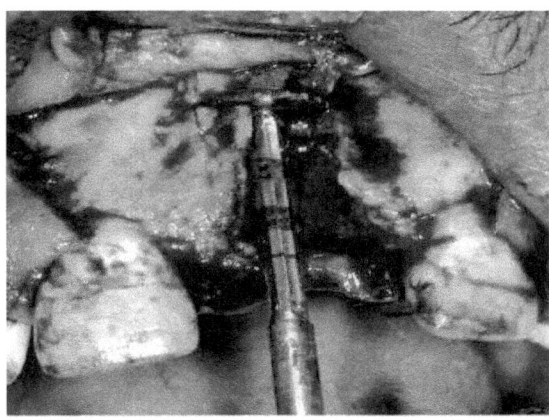

Lateral Cut Using Kc 7 And Lcd 7-4w

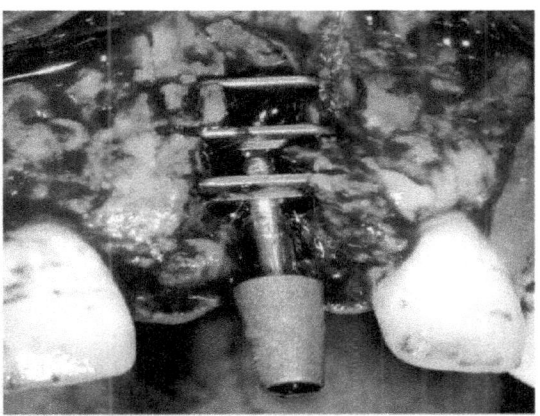

Insertion Of Boi, Bbbs 7

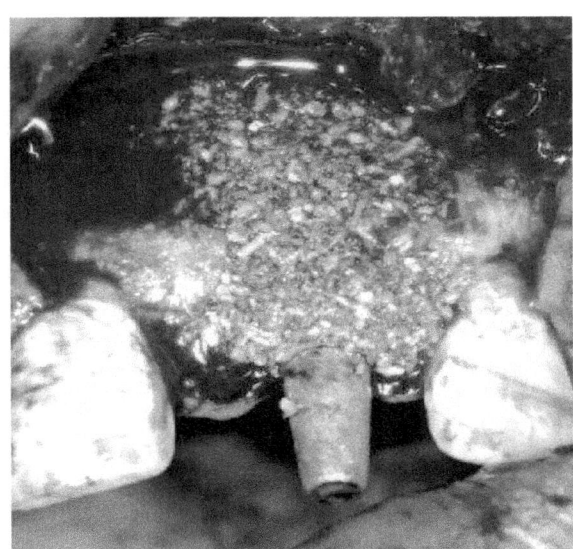

Placement of Particulate Bone Graft

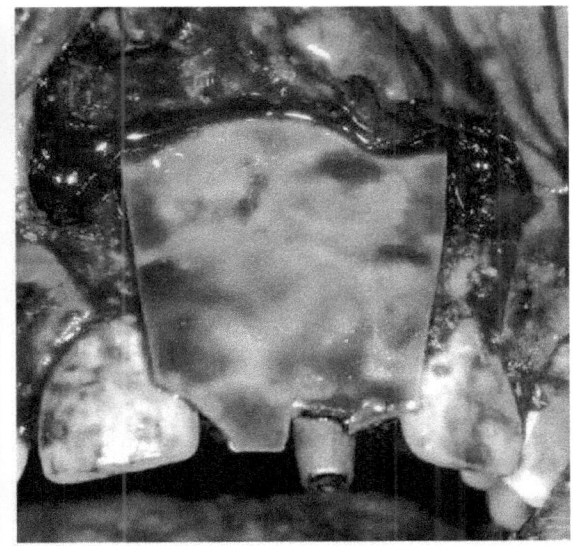

Placement of Resorbable Membrane

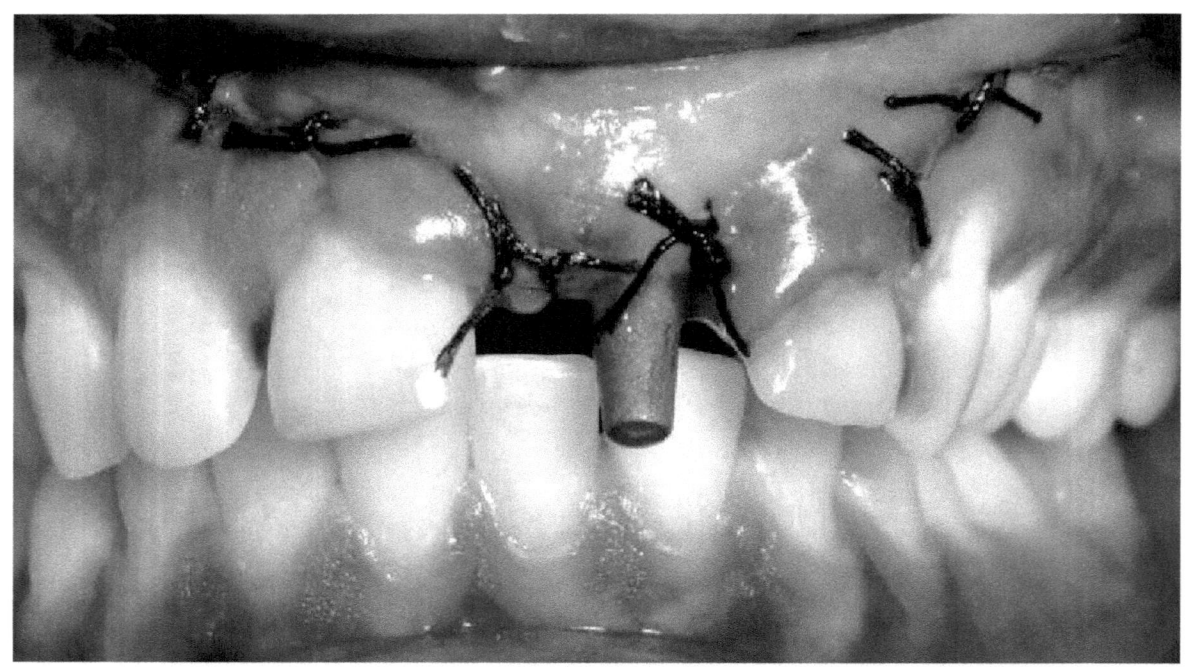

CLOSURE

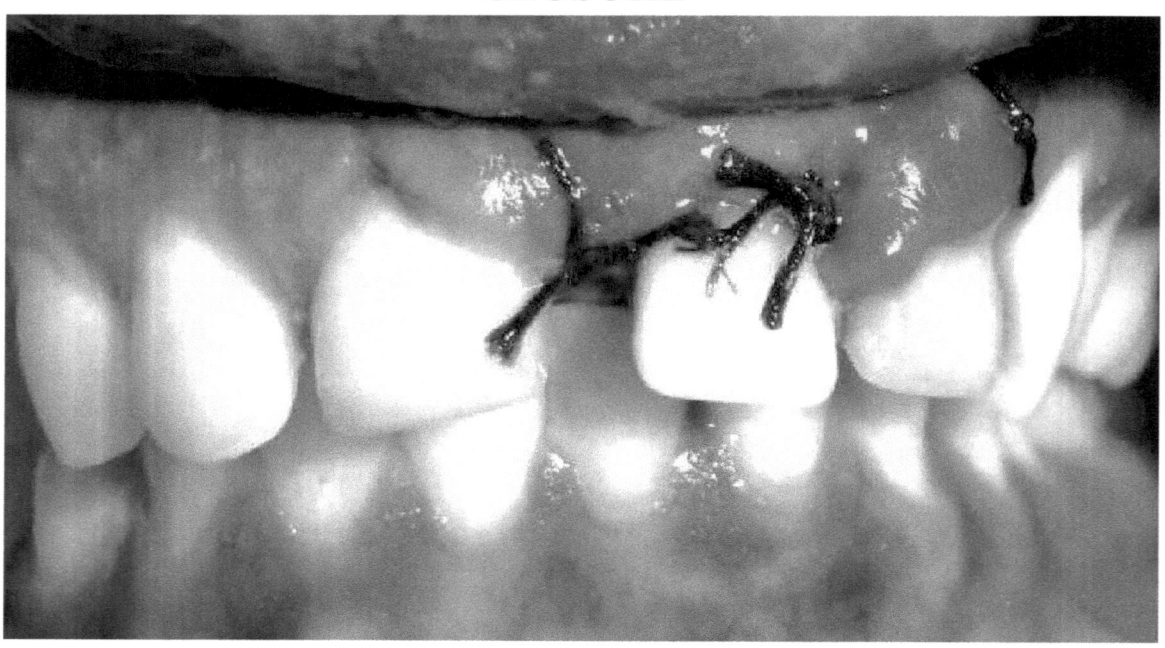

Immediate Restoration With Acrylic Crown

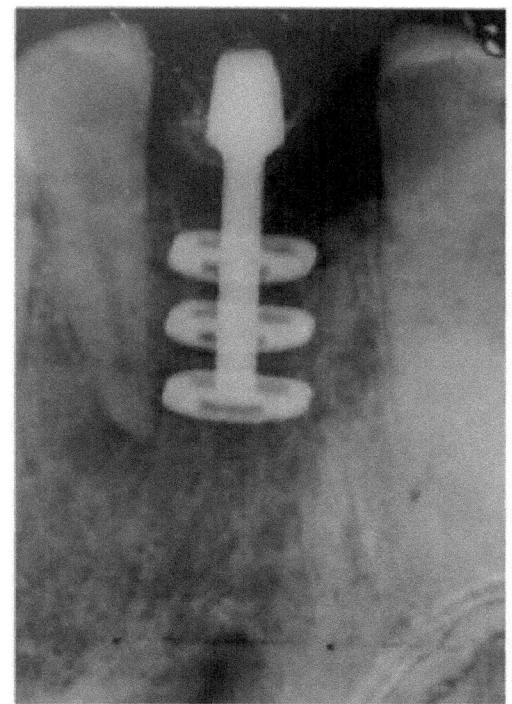 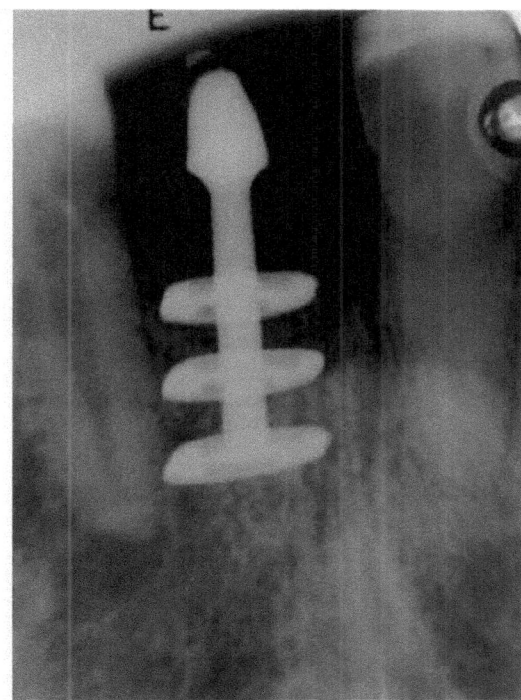

Immediate Post Operative Iopa   14 Months Post Operative Iopa

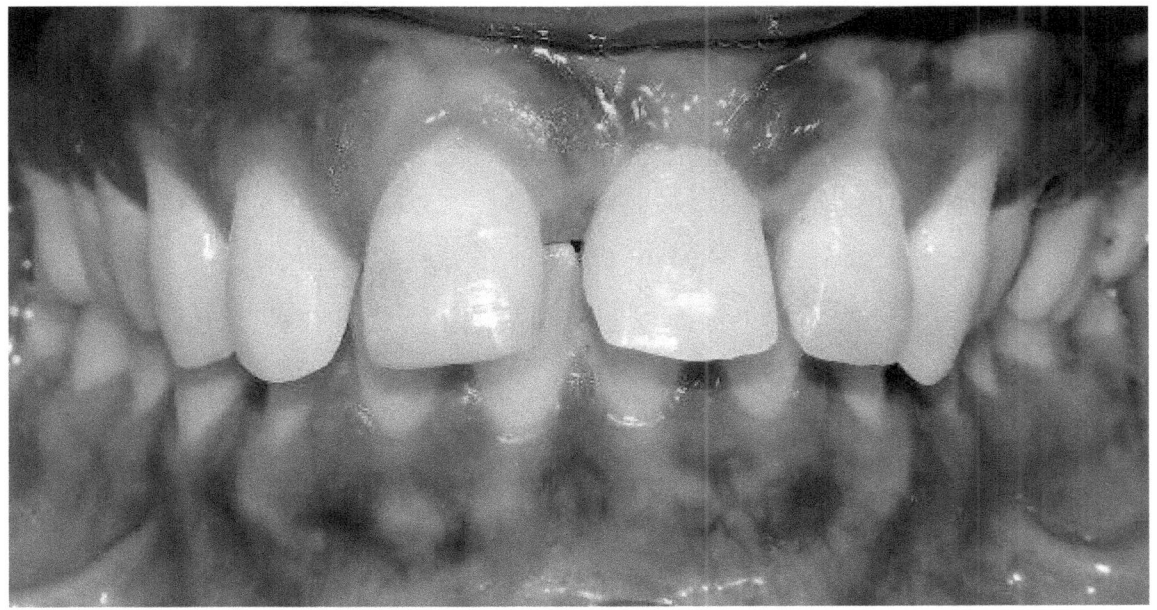

14 Months Post-Operative Photograph

Mandibular Posterior Boi Implant Placement

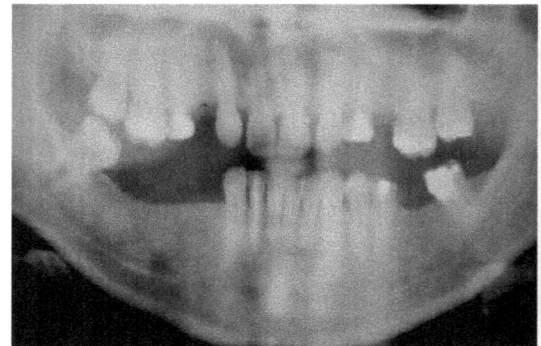

Pre-Operative Opg **Pre-Operative Photograph**

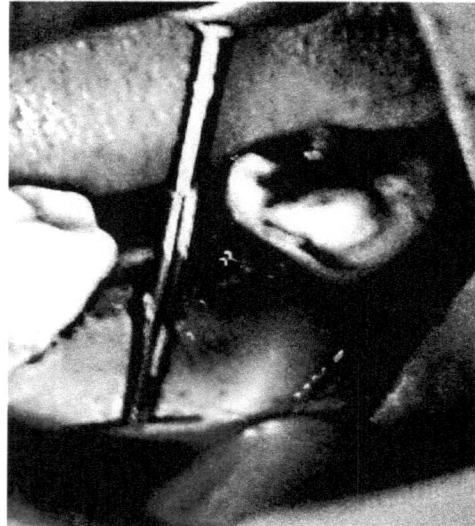
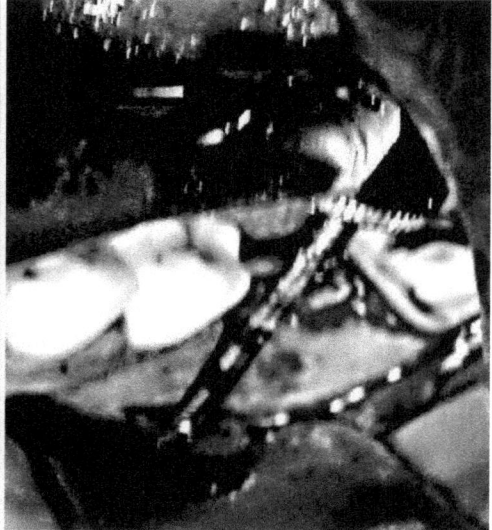

Vertical Cut Using Vc 1.6 Combination Cut Using Kc 7-4w

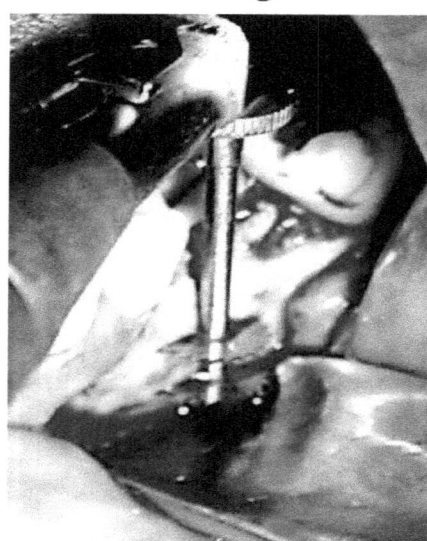
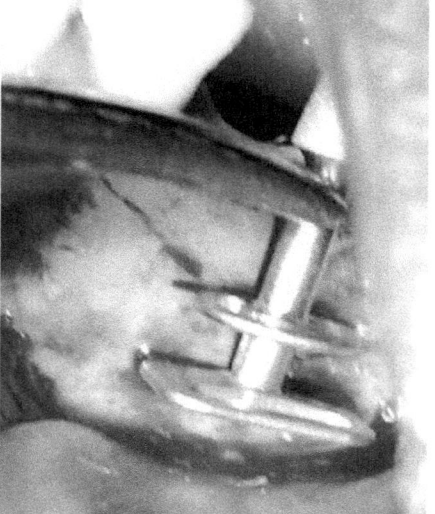

Lateral Cut Double Using Lcd 7-4w Placement Of Boi, BBS 9/7,H6

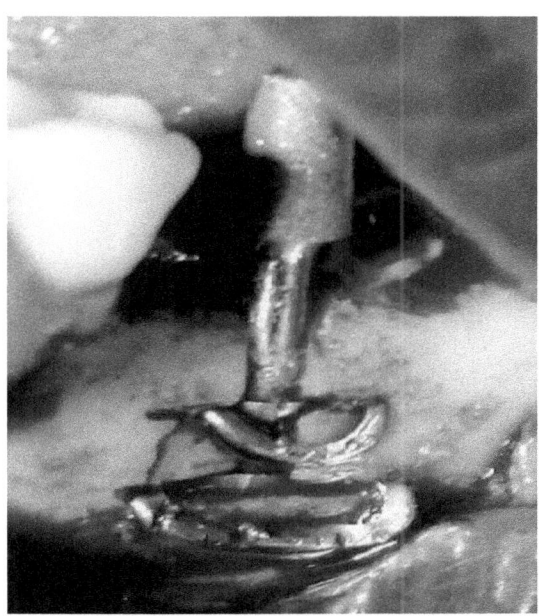

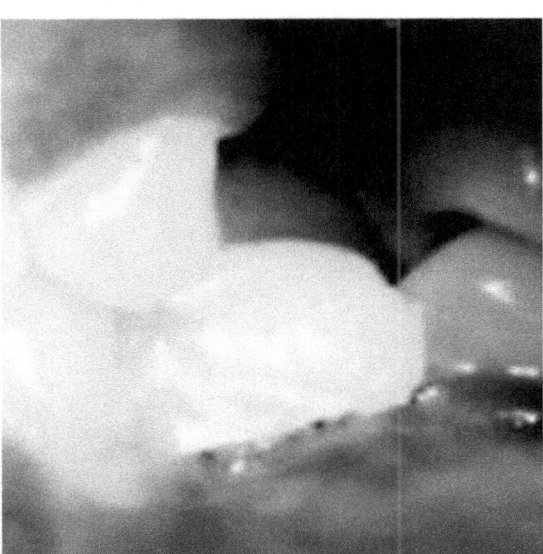

Immediate Restoration With Acrylic Crown

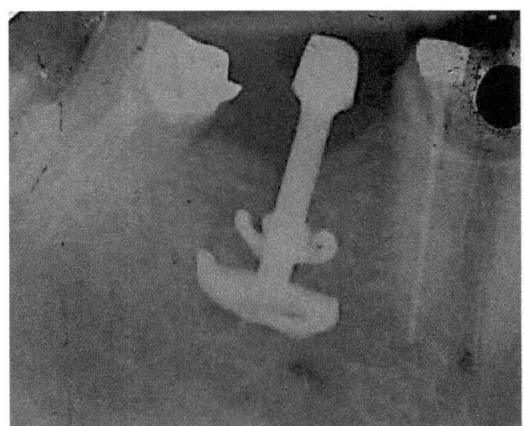
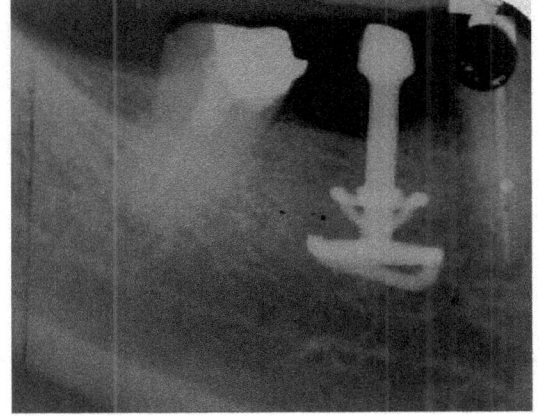

Immediate Post-Operative Iopa 14 Months Post-Operative Iopa

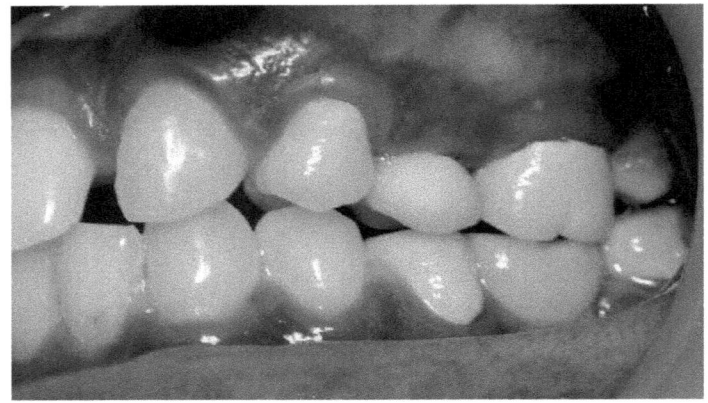

14 Months Post Operative Photograph With Ceramic Crown

Maxillary Anterior Boi Implant Placement In A Case Of Severe Bone Loss

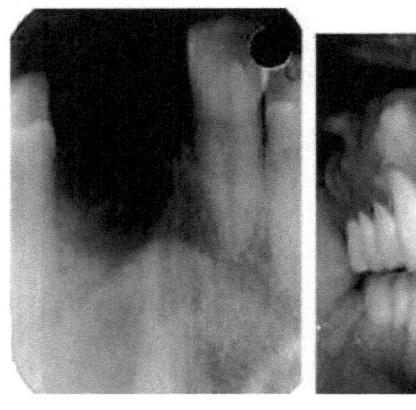 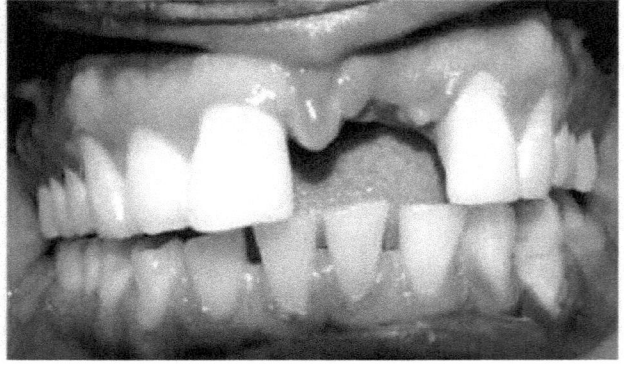

PREOP XRAY   **PREOPERATIVE PHOTOGRAPH**

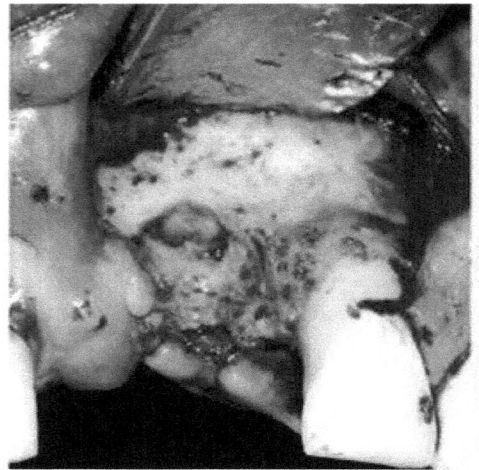 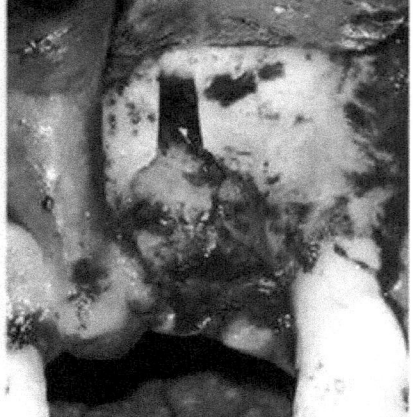

Surgical Exposur   **Osteotomy Done**

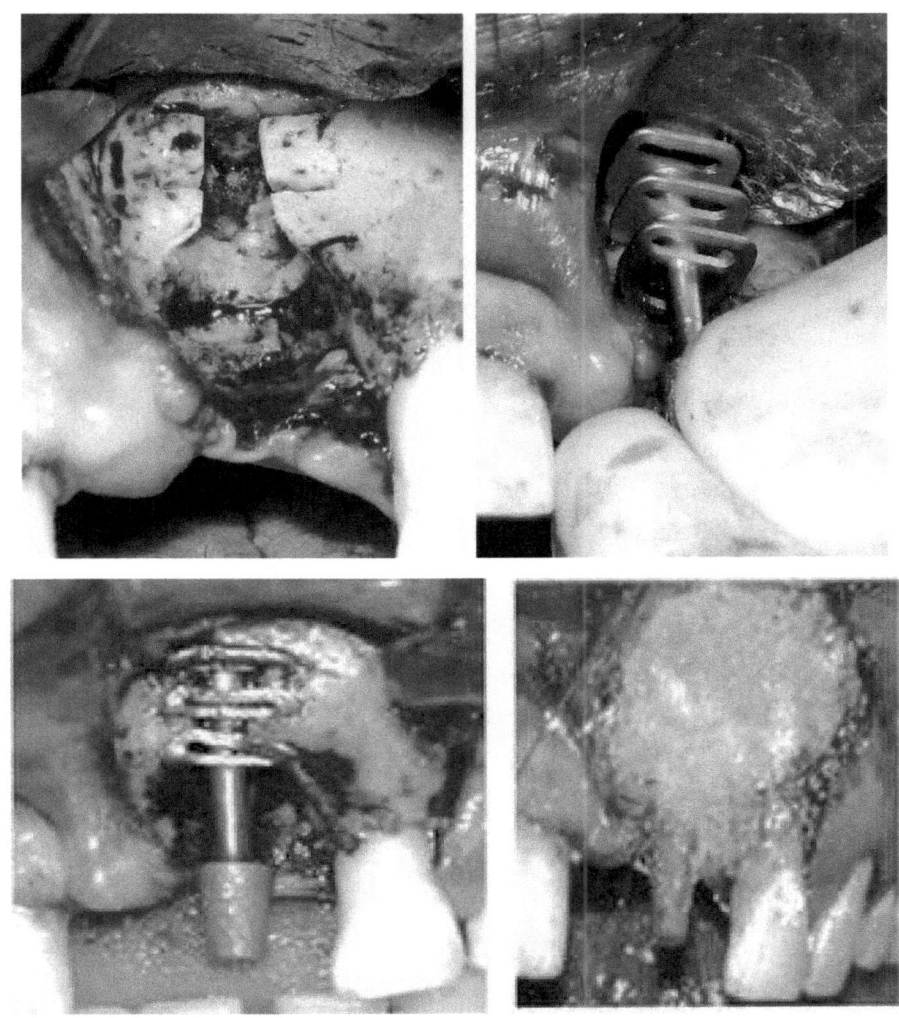

Implant Placement **Bone Graft Placed Along**

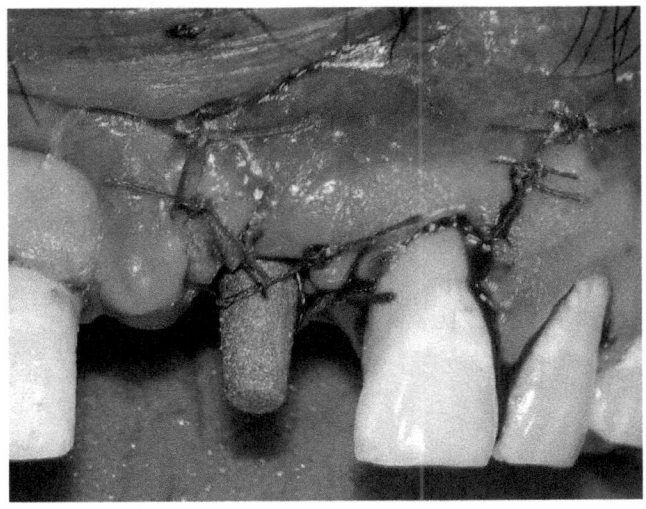

Suturing Done

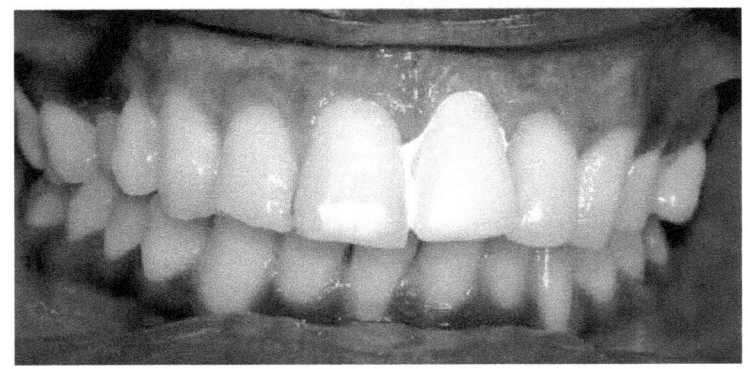

Temporization Done

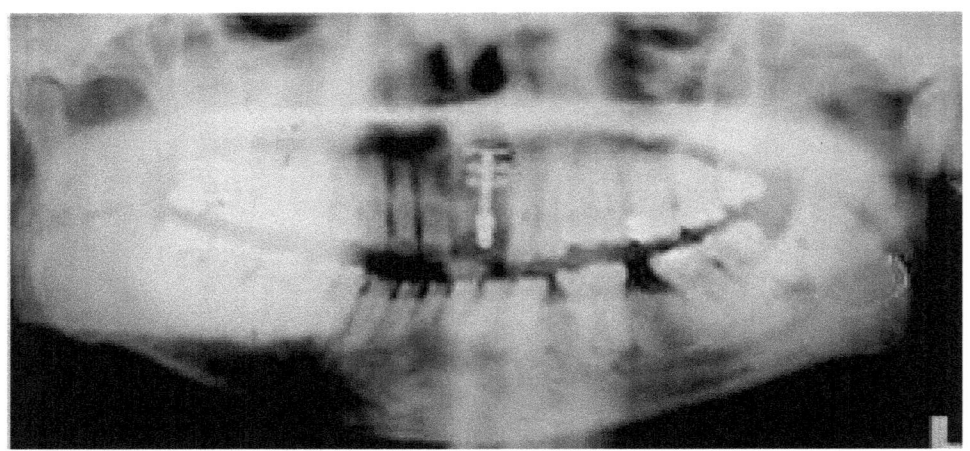

Post Operative Opg

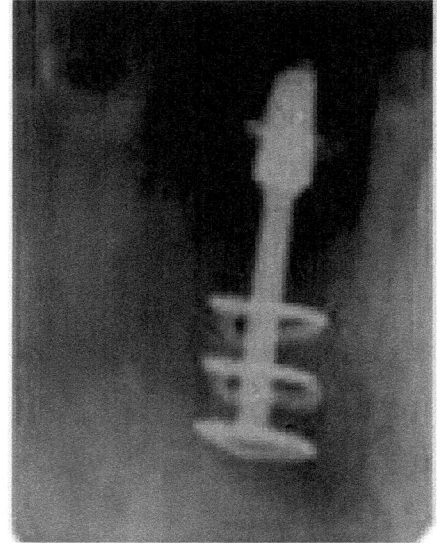

Post Operative Iopar

Discussion

Basal osseointegrated implants, offer an attractive alternative, even in small bone volumes, to conventional root-form implant placement, which often requires bone grafting [2].

Substantial implantological results can only be obtained if implants are incorporated intothe functional complex of the skull, do not affect the functional morphological changes of the jawbone[27]. Preferably they should be placed in areas where the bone is safe from resorption, so that enough volume will be available for many years to come. These safe regions include not only the mandibular anterior segment but other areas as well. BOI implant is a good alternative to crestal implants when additional procedures are indicated like in the region above the mandibular nerve, below the maxillary sinus, into extraction sockets of teeth, cavities and empty spaces left after cystectomies or granulation removals. After all lost bone structures will rebuild by themselves wherever functional loads induce them to rebuild or for that matter where the dentist indigenously directs them. The literature on basal implants had introduced the terms "Orthopaedic Technique" and "Orthopaedic Implant" to mark a clear distinction between them and the well known term "Dental Implant". They can be applied where very little vertical bone is present, while the supply of horizontal bone is still sufficient, even if these quantities are not contiguous such as in the sinus region. There are no difficult or impossible cases for implantologists familiar with basal implants, and their use leads in all cases straight forward to the desired treatment result[19].

Osseointegration with basal implants

During the insertion of basal implants, vertical and horizontal slots have to be prepared. The subsequent repair within the bone requires a complete remodelling of atleast the horizontal part of the mandible. These transosseous slots may be considered to be four semi fractures. Their repair leads to full remodeling of atleast the crestal horizontal part of mandible and this remodeling is accompanied with overall softening of bone[7].

The typical healing progression which follows is the the transformation of a blood clot to fibrous tissue, which later mineralizes and becomes woven bone. This woven bone may provide additional stabilization to the implant, although it continues to be remodeled over time into an even more supportive secondary osteonal bone, the end result of healing process[13].

These implants never experience Branemark style load transmission or osseointegration taking place along the vertical shaft of these designs.

An adequate blood supply is decisive for long term survival of BOI implants, which specifically applies to area of crestal disk as well. The BOI implants featuring larger disk to disk intervals of 5mm have found both basal plates integrated evenly well.

The formation of secondary osteons around one of the base plate does not seem to interfere with similar formations on the other basal plate. Also, the nutrient supply for each basal plate is assumed to be larger if the disks are located further apart. Problems with implant restoration systems supported by this type of implants are extremely rare.

Histologic proof of osseointegration of immediately loaded, laterally inserted disk type of implants was first obtained in 1985 when Juliet T3D titanium implant was removed from a patient prior to therapeutic irradiation.

Cortical bone has a very broad spectrum of functional adaptive mineralisations. Bicortical engagement of the base plate is mandatory in any case. Unicortically anchored disk implants have a high value of equivalent stress[8]. If double BOI implants are chosen, both base plates must be positioned below the white line[15]. The stress values are 15% lower in double disk implants than in single disk ones[10].

The stress is significantly lower during the complete osseointegration stage than during the stage when the implant is not integrated into the bone, that is after implant placement. Stress decreases by 10.1% in a stage of non- osseointegration, 28.8% in a stage between non-osseointegration and complete osseointegration, 58.4% when cortical bone grows into the implant body[11].

The maximum stress concentration is at the disc/shaft interface of the implant[3].

With the physiological stimulus by basal implants on present bone, remodeling leads to new vital bone in areas of load transmission[17].

The bone remodeling after surgery is in normal physiologic grade after about 1 year, so the influence of the factor of interest in this study is clearly distinguishable in this actual observation period.

Basal Implants Versus Crestal Implants

Survival rates for conventional dental implant systems are relatively high in normal healthy bone[16]. The management of poor bone with root form dental implants typically requires additional or augmentation procedures to ensure stability.

Disease, congenital anodontia, trauma or atrophy to the aging process leads to poor quality and quantity of bone[16]. Short implants are an alternative and yield acceptable results, as long as at least 5mm of vertical bone is available. However these implants cannot be used in immediate load procedures and due to their two-stage design the demand for attached gingiva in the mucosal penetration area and the demand for meticulous cleaning limits its use[14].

In addition traditional bullet shaped screw designs are not a option for treating such cases as these feature an internal screw connection, these require not only bone height, but also bone width. Their surface is roughened and the mucosal penetration diameter islarge. To prevent infections and bone loss, attached gingiva should surround the implant. Even if this is given, the effort for successful (professional and individual) cleaning is large because the sites are difficult to reach in cases of pronounced atrophy[14]. With basal implants degradation products of infection are resorbed via the periosteal tissues or removed to the oral cavity through the mucosal access. The necessary pressure is built from inside the bone. This pressure must never be blocked, and the direction of flow must never be inverted by the dentist. Early idiopathic lossthus hardly ever occurs with basal implants[19].

The very small demand for available bone qualifies BOI to be good for minimally invasive and fast treatment. Surface enhanced crestal implants are susceptible to peri- implantitis, which may lead to progressive ridge resorption. This is not present in basal implants because usually the disease stops as it reaches basal (resorption resistant) bone areas[19]. Also because of the narrow polished emergence of the implants and in addition the site of bacterial invasion is far away from site of force transmission, the bone is not burdened with two tasks at the same time. Moreover, the implant areas where the load transmission takes place are integrated in such a way that the osteogenic and osteoprotective properties of the cortical bone are utilized[27].

Scortecci et al. (2001) showed that 99% of the patients not eligible for treatment with screw implants can be treated by BOI without bone transplantation.

The vertical aspect of the cylindrical crestal implant must be placed in close contact to the alveolar bone for primary stability, a basal implant due to the nature of the insertion process, shows little or no contact in this area for some time[13].

Due to large support of the base plates, the dentist and the technician is allowed to take freedom in positioning of the masticatory surfaces, other than conventional implants, which are supported only by the bone near the vertical part of implant itself, and supporting polygon is reduced. Basal implants provide a wide and deep supporting polygon that provides good support to the prosthesis[15].

BOI in special situations
Vertical bone split procedures are useful if enough vertical bone is present pre - operatively, to insert at least short types of conventional implants.

Horizontal bone split procedures (distractions, bone interpositions) may also be used in order to increase bone volume. In cases of failure, the mobile crestal segment of the bone gets lost. Such patients can receive implants with an incomplete bi-cortical horizontal osteotomy allowing the insertion of the basal implant and immediate completion of the case without further necessity of increasing the bone volume, transporting bone, a second stage surgery, etc[14].

With basal implants, augmentatioin and reopening is avoided, they have immediate function and are generally implanted simultaneously with extraction16. There has been a success rate of 98.1% for basal implants in fresh extraction sockets even after 4.5 years[22].

Patients who have been treated successfully with implants in the past, will likely select implants in lieu of prosthesis, in the event of an implant failure. Use of BOI implants in such patients can avoid the long waiting periods associated with other modes of restoring the normal masticatory function[9]. Also when conventional dental implant systems fail, there is typically little bone for immediate re-implantation. For BOI implants, almost any amount of bone remaining is sufficient for corrective procedures in most cases. This coupled with the patient benefit of immediate functional use makes BOI an excellent alternative for treating patient with failed dental implants.

Basal implants are not known to show crater-like bone defects, possibly due polished vertical implant surface area[13].

If the patient suffers from osteoporosis, basal implants may be placed in the manner of subperiosteal implants. Implants with length of 33 and 43 mm are available. Thediameter of the central base plate is 9mm[14].

Smokers and non-smokers experience similar rate of implant losses. This may indicate that smokers, reported as having a higher risk of implant loss than the conventional implants may benefit from BOI implant treatment[16]. It is however, recommended that, patients should not smoke for atleast 6 weeks before and 3 weeks after the procedure[27].

Periodontal diseases are generally considered to be a contraindication for implantologists even if revitalized. The presence of germs and a history of ineffective treatments give a difficult prognosis for crestal implants[18]. The advantage of basal implants is the dysjunction of the infection risk area of gum perforation and the load transmitting areas in the aseptic deep basal cortical bone. Even in cases where BOI"sare immediately inserted into the infected alveoli, the healing can"t be disturbed by infection and functional load[18]. The first reason are the horizontal osteotomy cuts in the deepest area where a wound drain is not hindered as typical with screw type implants, sealing bone hermitically. Second, the geometry of BOI is infection preventive. The thin, smooth vertical shaft (diameter < 2mm), is not directly load transmitting to the crestal bone. So plaque and calculus adherence is rare and far away from force fit implant interaction. Mucositis linked with BOI is reported rarely (<1%).

Design and selection of basal implants

The only statistically significant factor on success is the implant design. Studies have shown that, survival rate in multiple disk implants (96.6%), is 1.7% higher than those with single disk (94.9%)[16].

In BOI systems, the fate of the alveolar ridge is not linked to the fate of the implant-restoration complex, since the areas where load transmission takes place are spatially separated from masticatory surfaces. This fact is obvious from the design of BOI implants[27].

The crestal and basal plates of the multi-disk BOI inplant restoration systems have different functions. The main purpose of the crestal plate is to provide additionalstabilization of the implant. The crestal plate loses its importance once the basal plate has ossified to full load bearing capacity. The web-bar of the crestal plate is located perpendicular to the web bars of the basal plate. In other words, this part of the crestal plate is inserted directly into the palatal bone well protected against resorption.

The osteotomy area in the vestibular bone is crossed only by the ring of the crestal plate. The ring acts like a tent keeping the periosteum away from the bone, thus facilitating any primary or secondary augmentation procedures.

Multiple disk implants are used in higher but narrow bone (canine eminence, anterior alveolar ridge) single disk implants when vertical bone loss is extreme (sinus region, above the mandibular canal), so leverage differences are obvious[16].

Double or multiple disk implants have been available in France since around 1988. The disk to disk interval on these implants is 3mm. specific double cutters matching these distances for lateral osteotomy are available. Also implants and osteotomy tools for 5mm disk to disk, intervals are also available.

The rectangular design of the disks is flattened on one side and remain rounded on the other side. The rectangular side faces the vestibular aspect and the rounded side remains on the medial aspect. This led to the main burden of load shifted to the vestibular bone. Some users have modified this and inserted the other way where the main burden of load transmission is shifted to the medial bone structure as the vestibular bone structure is charecterized by extreme resorption

The diameter of the basal disk in BOI implants should be as large as possible to meet prosthetic requirements. From the BOI implantologists view point, implants featuring a load-transmitting basal plate of less than 9mm in diameter (particularly those with a thickness of 0.6mm or more) must be regarded as rigid implants with a larger disk diameter are more elastic than with a smaller diameter disk of same thickness. The load transmitting surfaces of these implants are located farther away from potential infection entry points. This after all is the ultimate criterion for long term survival of the implants.

The distance between the load transmitting surfaces and the site of bacterial attack can be increased by using a large-diameter disk. An alternative option would be to select an implant with a longer shaft.

The web bars connect the disk of the vertical shaft. The shape and size of these bars depends on their function of converting functional loads to isoelastic vibrations and cyclic loads that the supporting bone can tolerate.

The bars should be resilient to fracture and capable of force distribution over larger bone areas to avoid osteolysis by local stress concentrations.

An equilibrated masticatory pattern is of particular importance for maintaining mineralization in the interfacial region, especially in the first months after implant placement[19]. Only when bilaterally identical AFMP (Planas" Masticatory Functional Angle) is present, the chewing activity of the patient will be equal on both sides. Often too long vestibular cusps in the upper jaw are the reason for non-identical angles[18].

Masticatory forces transmitted via the basal implants to an enossal location create local microcracks in the cortical bone as described earlier . Microcracks are replaced by the formation of secondary osteons, a process called remodeling. This however, will temporarily increase the porosity of the affected bone region and temporarily reduce the degree of mineralization additionally. Basal implants in this status have a good chance of getting reintegrated at a high degree of mineralization, if loads are reduced to an adequate amount[19].

BOI in posterior maxilla

Maxillary sinus elevation and bone augmentation are acceptable techniques that may provide sufficient bone quantity and quality for implant support in the posterior atrophic maxilla. However given the risk of morbidity along with the cost and time consuming effects, these techniques are to be reconsidered. Simpler and safer protocols are therefore required for the posterior maxilla, where bone resorption, deficient posterior alveolar ridge andincreased pneumatisation of the sinus, all result in a minimal hard tissue bed thus rendering implant placement difficult[1]

The conditions in the maxilla regarding the relationship between internal pressure and external (that is cortical) compressive/tensile stresses are not the same as in mandible.In these cases, greater number of disks per implant should be selected. Also combination with several crestal implants may be desirable to ensure adequate stability of the structure.

Single base plate implants may be placed under the sinus in as little as 3mm vertical bone height, utilizing stable cortical anchoring. We have observed an good primary stability for placement and immediate restoration with BOI implant sub-antrally and also trans-antrally.

The BOI implants have a smooth shaft, without causing any noticeable irritation for bacterial inoculation. Also it makes the implant restoration complex more elastic. This structural detail prepared the ground for comprehensive implant therapy along the maxillary sinus, by placing the disk and the shaft inside the sinus.

BOI in posterior mandible

For placing basal implants crestal to the nerve in the posterior mandible, approximately 2-3 mm of vertical bone above the alveolar nerve is necessary and the morphology of the bone must allow the insertion of a bicortically anchored base plate and cover it as much as possible[14]. The base plates of these implants is generally 0.7mm high and at the top of the base plate another 1-2 mm of native bone should be available[14]. However careful placement and advanced experience are required as there is anecdotal evidence that some of the attached complications to using basal implants can be fracture of implant, iatrogenic mandibular fracture and advanced nerve sensation[14].

The atrophic bone in distal jaws is frequently broad, which is an ideal condition for basal implants due to their lateral placement[16].

Posterior implants in mandible are usually square- shaped having a disc of 9x12mm, 9x16mm, 10x14mm with shafts of 6-13.5mm in length, depending on the desired vertical dimension and available horizontal bone. The thickness of the base plate itself is 0.6-0.9 mm, allowing the implant to participate in the flexion of the mandible and provides safe ground for fixed prosthesis[15].

Failure to place the distal BOI implant below the white line will result in loss of bone (due to overload osteolysis, often combined with an infection) and subsequently in the loss of the implant[15].

Also, placement of BOI in posterior mandible was found to be more technically demanding due to the thick nature of the cortical bone, which does not give way to minor adjustments as possible in the porous bone of the maxilla.

BOI in aesthetic zone

When teeth in aesthetic zone are scheduled for extraction and replacement by implants, this poses a combination of challenges. First it is often difficult to anchor conventional implants because the buccopalatal and the mesiodistal dimensions of the tooth roots are greater than the dimensions of the implants. Further, we have experienced cases with loss of labial cortical plate in the central incisor region. In such cases cases, the use of a multi-disk BOI implant with the most basal disk inserted into the thick cortical bone below the anterior nasal spine is a good option. In addition intense bone remodeling and soft tissue recontouring occur, which make it difficult to achieve a lasting aesthetic result quickly. A combination of a single-stage surgical approach with a two-stage prosthetic approach is one option to solve this problem[6]. Augmentation may still be necessary in aesthetic zones. The vestibular struts of BOI implants may project out of the bone and support the augmentation material. In this technique, augmentation may be performed simultaneously with implant placements. The decrease in total treatment time may reach upto 98% [24].

DO'S and DONT'S with BOI

Examining the status of the peri-implant bone is considered malpractice with basal implants, as no osseointegration is required on the vertical aspect of the implant anyway for permanent function of the implant[19].

Probing may carry pathogens to the depths of the interfacial region that is filled with non-irritant connective tissue at a time when there is little chance of suppuration left. Callus formation and the maturation of the callus in the slot areas are endangered through probing. Facultative pathogens can be transported to an environment, that is normally inaccessible to them and cause great damage. In particular, the maxillary sinusarea may be contaminated by germs of oral - origin by simple probing, if bone height is reduced or if a trans-sinus insertion was performed. Probing around basal implants is therefore contraindicated and is potentially dangerous[19].

Anterior patterns of chewing are to be avoided. These patterns lead to an extrusion of implants in the posterior segments and at the same time the bone area around the implants are subject to tensile forces, which reduce the mineralization significantly[15].

When approaching from the vestibular side, the facial artery and its vein must be protected meticulously with the help of a broad spatula or an instrument in the shape of a soup spoon[14].

Reasons for failure of the implants are poor oral hygiene, poor bone quality, compromised medical status of the patient and biomechanical factors. Various authors have stressed the importance of biomechanical factors such as type of loading, the bone implant interface, the length and diameter of implants, shape and chareteristics of implant surface, the prosthesis type and the quantity and again the quality of surrounding bone[3].

Implant displacement within the bone depends simply on the degree of osseointegration[10].

Osseointegration at a lowered degree of mineralization is not the same as "fibrointegration". Orthopaedic surgeons describe the equivalent status of orthopaedic implants as "sterile loosening", but they have no means of treating the status. Basal implants in this status have good chance of getting reintegrated at a high degree of mineralization, if loads are reduced to an adequate amount[19]. For sterile loosening of basal implants, numerous therapeutic options exist; functional adjustment or combined surgical/functional treatment of bone/implant/restoration systems are required and in some cases the reduction of muscle forces is part of the therapy plan. Such options are not given for crestal implants. Even the replacement or addition of basal implants is easily possible, since there is usually sufficient cortical bone available for additive therapy[19].

If an indication for replacing basal implant really exists, this measure should be taken right away, since mobile implants will invariably cause bone damage. By contrast with screw type implants, BOI implants will never exfoliate spontaneously. For this reason and because overload trauma may be transferred from one side of the jaw to the other via the denture or via a involuntary change in the preferred working side, there is no point waiting.

The objective of any replacement will be to restore the full function of the fixed restoration and thereby the full range of masticatory movements. This is why the insertion of the new implant must be planned along with the removal of old implant. In most cases immediate reimplantation will be possible and indicated. Problems must be addressed immediately and professionally, not least in order to prevent the spread of overload related damage to other implants, which carries a risk of subsequent fracture and overload osteolysis and thus to prevent bone loss. It is not necessary to wait with corrective intervention, because every patient has enough bone for treatment with basal implants[19].

Survival data of BOI

Basal implants used for single tooth replacement showed the lowest survival rate (90.9%) by Kopp, but this was result of specific overload due to non-physiologic, uncompensated forces[23].

The better survival rates in implants longer in situ comes from their survival of initial threats as possible infections, malocclusions and surgical and prosthodontics mistakes[16].

Donsimoni et al. reported a 97% survival rate and a 100% clinical success rate. Similar results have been reported by Scortecci, Kopp, Ihde and Mutter and Ihde. However this was with the use of basal osseointegrated implants which were always splinted with other implants (basal or crestal implants) or with natural teeth.

The quality of life, was ultimately evaluated by the ability to chew all range of foods native to the diet, to speak legibly, socially acceptable smile and dentofacial profile and comfortable without halitosis and pain. Various studies shows a good success rate in use of these implants for single & multiple tooth replacements, however a larger group of patients need to be evaluated to generalize the data.

Summary And Conclusion

The standard procedure for placing basal implants includes one surgery followed by immediately loading, thus reducing time, cost and stress to the patient. With the emphasis on horizontal rather than vertical placement, pre-implantological bone augmentation was never required for anchorage.

Primary stability is never an issue with basal osseointegrated implants because of the implant design and bicortical nature of anchorage. This offers several advantages like - no hospitalization required, no time period with loss of esthetics and a missing tooth, low degree of invasiveness, no second surgery, no bone transplants, no bone distractions, simple repair in difficult areas, manageable system (few components), simple lab technique.

However, stock keeping requirements are greater than in basal implantology. It will always be necessary to keep a few more implants handy to avoid extensive planning including three dimensional exploration of bone conditions.

Also, the technique poses substantial challenges for instructors and users alike, as far as the surgical and prosthetic treatment stages and substantial knowledge requirements in the field of biomechanics and bone physiology are concerned.

Basal implants have always shown to perform well in immediate load conditions, when splinted with other implants or natural teeth. But when they are subjected to a loading protocol which is gradual and not immediate, it does not seem to affect the osseointegraton, insingle tooth edentulous sites. Immediate restoration in such cases would not significantly increase the load over the implant during this period. Mild contacts during mastication though unavoidable, acts like a stimulation for bone remodeling to take place.

Various authors have observed a good success rate in the implant. Although, a larger sample size is required to generalize this data.

All studies reached and maintained the treatment aim of immediate restoration and early occlusal loading. This indicates that, placement of basal osseointegrated implants in single & multiple edentulous sites is a predictable and reliable procedure and is a good option to be considered in compromised situations to avoid additional procedures like bone grafting and sinus lifts.

Bibliography

1. Adel A Chidiac: Safe and effective alternatives to sinus elevation in atrophied posterior maxilla.

   Implants; 2010: 1: 6-10.

2. Gerard Scortecci: Immediate function of cortically anchored disk-design implants without bone augmentation in moderately to severely resorbed completely edentulous maxillae.

   Journal of Oral Implantology; 1999: 25: 70-79.

3. Goldman T, Ihde S : Stress distribution within basal dental implants and on the interface to the bone. Influence of the design of the bridgework in the atrophied posterior mandible: the concept of the supporting polygon. Craniomaxillofacial Implant Directions; 2011: 6: 43-56.

4. Guillaume Odin, Thierry Balaguer, Charles Savoldelli, Gerard Scortecci: Immediate functional loading of an implant-supported fixed prosthesis at the time of ablative surgery and mandibular reconstruction for squamous cell carcinoma.

   Journal of Oral Implantology; 2010: 36: 225-230.

5. Henri Diederich: Immediate loading of maxillary full arch rehabilitation supported by basal and crestal implants. Craniomaxillofacial Implant Directions; 2008: 3: 61-63.

6. Henri Diederich: Immediately loaded maxillary reconstruction using basal and crestal implants, with delayed esthetic adaptation of the bridgework. Craniomaxillofacial Implant Directions; 2007: 2: 161-164.

7. Ihde S, Himmlova L, Tomas Goldmann: Post-operative remodeling of the mandibular bone allows the incorporation of stiff circular bridges on four strategically placed basal implants in an immediate load protocol. Craniomaxillofacial Implant Directions; 2011: 6: 57-67.

8. Ihde Stefan K.A, Vitomir S. Konnstantinovic: Immediate loading of Dental Implants: Where is the dip ? Craniomaxillofacial Implant Directions; 2007: 2:145-154.

9. Ihde Stefan K.A: BOI a case of immediate loading alternative after failed dental implants. Craniomaxillofacial Implant Directions; 2007: 2: 72-77.

10. Libor Borak, Peter Marcian, Zdenek Florian, Sonia Bartakova: Biomechanical study of disk implants – Part I Engineering Mechanics;2010: 17: 49-60.

11. Petr Marcian, Zdenek Florian, Libor Borak, David Krpalek, Jırı Valasek: Biomechanical study of disk implants – Part II Engineering Mechanics; 2010: 17: 111-121.

12. Ruzov E, Ihde A: Flap closure technique for single-piece, lateral basal implants. Craniomaxillofacial Implant Directions; 2011: 6: 20-25.

13. Stefan Ihde, Tomas Goldmann, Lucie Himmlova, Zoran Aleksic, Gommiswald: The use of finite element analysis to model bone-implant contact with basal implants. Oral Surg Oral Med Oral Pathol Oral Radiol Endod; 2008: 106: 39-48.

14. Stefan K.A. Ihde, Vitomior S. Konstantinovic, Ihde Antonina A: Restoring the severely atrophied posterior mandible with basal implants: A comparison of four different surgical approaches. Craniomaxillofacial Implant Directions; 2011:6: 3-18.

15. Siddharth Shah: Strategic implant placement – Basal implants below theamber line (linea obliqua) in mandible. Craniomaxillofacial Implant Directions; 2011: 6: 33-41

16. Sigmar Kopp: Basal implants: A safe and effective treatment option in dental implantology. Craniomaxillofacial Implant Directions; 2007: 3:110-117.

17. Sigmar Kopp: Implantological treatment in a patient with hypodontia. Craniomaxillofacial Implant Directions; 2007: 2: 155-159.

18. Sigmar Kopp: "All on four"- basal implants as solid base for circularbridges in high periodontal risk patients.

    Craniomaxillofacial Implant Directions; 2007: 3: 105-108.

19. Stefan Ihde: Comparison of Basal and Crestal implants and their modus ofapplication. Smile Dental Journal; 2009: 4: 36-46.

20. Stefan Ihde, Sigmar Kopp: No More Sinus Lifts- Application of concepts steaming from orthopedic surgery for effective dental implant procedures in the distal maxilla. Smile Dental Journal; 2010: 5: 14-21

21. Stefan Ihde, Sigmar Kopp, Antonina Ihde: Palatal insertion of basal implants: case report and discussion of an alternative technique of maxillary implant placement. Smile Dental Journal; 2010: 5: 20-25.

22. Sigmar Kopp: Full mouth rehabilitation – from extraction to full arch bridges in just one day. Craniomaxillofacial Implant Directions; 2008: 3:191-200.

23. Sigmar Kopp: Basal implants: A safe and effective option in dental implantology. Craniomaxillofacial Implant Directions; 2007: 3: 111-118.

24. Stefan Ihde, Sigmar Kopp, Thomas Maier: Comparison of implant survival with implants placed in acceptable and compromised bone: aliterature review. J. Maxillofac Oral Surg; 2009: 8: 1-7

25. Sigmar Kopp, Wilfried Kopp: Comparison of Immediate Vs delayed basal implants. Journal of Maxillofacial and Oral Surgery; 2008: 7: 116-122

26. Sigmar Kopp, Halina Panek, Stefan Ihde, Bela Lieb: Clinical Problems with Implant Installation in Geriatic Patients. Dent. Med. Probl; 2009: 46:486-493

27. Stefan Ihde (2004) : Principles of BOI – Clinical, Scientific and Practical Guidelines to 4-D Dental Implantology; Springer Verlag Berlin Heidelberg.

28. Vitomir S Konstantinovic, Vojkan Lazic, Stefan Ihde: The nasal epithesis retained by basal (disk) implants.Journal of Craniofacial Surgery; 2010: 21: 33-36